Praise for

THE FIRST YEAR®

Hepatitis C

"The authors, who are both infected with hepatitis C (HCV), add to Marlowe's 'First Year' series for new patients with a how-to-respond guide that moves from the day of diagnosis through the first year of coping. HCV, a blood-borne virus, infects nine million Americans and nearly 200 million people worldwide. Even so, the general public remains unaware that this chronic illness is epidemic and that there is no effective treatment for the majority of its victims. The good news, as this book makes clear, is that HCV can be managed. In this straightforward, day-by-day manual, the authors provide a schedule for learning just about everything one needs to know about living with 'hep C.'"

—*Library Journal*

CARA BRUCE is a freelance writer who has edited four books and coauthored one. Her articles have appeared in *The San Francisco Bay Guardian*, Salon.com, *Maxim*, and dozens of other publications. Her fiction has appeared in numerous magazines, Web sites, and anthologies, including *Best American Erotica 2001* (Simon & Schuster) and *Pills, Chills, and Thrills* (Alyson Books 2004).

LISA MONTANARELLI is the coauthor of three books. Her articles have appeared in *Art and Antiques, The History Channel Magazine, San Francisco Chronicle* and *Publishers Weekly*, and her fiction has been published in *Best American Erotica 2004* and *Best American Erotica 2005* (Simon & Schuster). She has a B.A. from Yale and a Ph.D. in Comparative Literature from U.C. Berkeley. Visit her at LisaMontanarelli.com.

THE FIRST YEAR®

Hepatitis C

An Essential Guide for the Newly Diagnosed

Second Edition, Completely
Revised and Updated

Cara Bruce and
Lisa Montanarelli

MARLOWE & COMPANY ■ NEW YORK

THE FIRST YEAR®—*HEPATITIS C Second Edition:*
An Essential Guide for the Newly Diagnosed
Copyright © 2002, 2007 by Lisa Montanarelli and Cara Bruce
Foreword copyright © 2002 by Teresa L. Wright, M.D.

Published by
Marlowe & Company
An Imprint of Avalon Publishing Group, Incorporated
11 Cambridge Center
Cambridge, MA 02142

AVALON
publishing group incorporated

The First Year® is a trademark of
the Avalon Publishing Group.

The Library of Congress has catalogued the previous edition as follows:
Library of Congress Cataloging-in-Publication
Montanarelli, Lisa.
    The first year—hepatitis C : an essential guide for the newly
diagnosed / Lisa Montanarelli and Cara Bruce ; foreword by
Teresa Wright
        p. cm.
    Includes bibliographical references and index.
    ISBN 1-56924-541-X
    1. Hepatitis C—Popular works. I. Bruce, Cara. II. Title.

RC848.H425 M66 2002
616,3'623—dc21

                                    2001055871

ISBN 10: 1-60094-028-5
ISBN 13: 978-1-60094-028-6

9 8 7 6 5 4 3 2 1

Designed by Pauline Neuwirth,
    Neuwirth and Associates, Inc.

Printed in the United States of America

To our families, Paul, Diane
and Alli Bruce and Stephen
and Jane Montanarelli.
They have given us
the most invaluable help of all.

Contents

Contents

Foreword

by Teresa L. Wright, M.D.

THERE HAS been increased awareness about hepatitis C (HCV) over the past decade, so that HCV is now being described as "the new HIV." While it is likely that for many years, HCV did not receive the public attention or funding that it deserved, and while it is promising that public education has improved in recent years, it is also important that we put hepatitis C in perspective with other public health problems.

Hepatitis C is much more common than HIV (infecting three to four times as many individuals in the U.S. alone). HCV is transmitted in similar ways to HIV, through blood exposures, from contaminated needles, and occasionally from high-risk sexual exposure. Like HIV, HCV is an RNA virus that changes over time and that would be predicted to evade the immune response and rapidly to develop resistance to treatments. Like HIV, there is no effective vaccine against HCV, nor is there likely to be one in the foreseeable future. Like HIV, HCV is common in underserved communities—the homeless, people in prison, minority populations, veterans.

However, HCV and HIV are very different in terms of the diseases that result from long-standing infection. They are also different in the ease by which they are transmitted sexually—HIV can be readily transmitted through unprotected sex, HCV much less so. They differ in our ability to treat these infections, with many more drugs available for treatment of HIV infection than for HCV. The natural history of HCV and HIV are both variable. Some people can be infected for many years without serious consequences, and others develop progressive disease over a decade (or in the case of HIV, over even shorter periods). However, untreated HIV infection is much more likely to result in life-threatening complications and debilitating disease than is untreated HCV infection. Indeed the majority of those with HCV infection will never develop advanced liver disease or liver cancer. Short of these severe complications, patients with HCV may have reduced quality of life or symptoms from involvement of organs outside of the liver. This impaired quality of life sometimes improves with therapy.

Patients should take heart from the slow natural history of HCV infection. If they either cannot tolerate current medications, or have failed current medications, particularly if they have mild liver damage as shown from a liver biopsy, patients should focus on living a long and active life with hepatitis C, rather than focus on the potential for their disease to progress.

Of course, there are certain populations with hepatitis C that particularly require active and aggressive treatment if available. These include (i) patients with stage III or stage IV scarring to the liver; (ii) patients who have developed complications of their liver disease such as liver failure, fluid in the belly (ascites), changed mental function (encephalopathy) and internal bleeding (variceal bleeding); (iii) patients with HIV co-infection, since advance liver disease appears most common in this group and since many cannot tolerate their HIV medications because of their liver disease; (iv) patients following liver transplantation who have already experienced life-threatening complications of HCV infection and who are at risk for losing their new liver from further infection; (v) and, finally, patients with HCV-related hepatocellular carcinoma in whom treatment options are limited.

Cara Bruce and Lisa Montanarelli's *The First Year®—Hepatitis C* will be an excellent resource for all patients with hepatitis C infection, whether they are patients with no symptoms at all but are worried about giving HCV infection to their loved ones; whether they have mild liver disease but have fatigue that is affecting their daily lives; or whether they have some of the complications of long-standing HCV infection described above. HCV, like

HIV, is an infection that people have to live with, often for many, many years. To this end, patients need practical common-sense advice about diet, exercise, modification of lifestyles and dealing with the depression that comes from living with a chronic illness. Cara Bruce and Lisa Montanarelli provide a comprehensive guide to help the patient with all aspect of hepatitis C infection. Their advice is essential, since most doctors focus mainly on the medical aspects of this disease with their patients. There is obviously much more information needed to help patients live long and productive lives. For a few, HCV infection will be treated and cured. For the majority, either because treatments haven't worked, or more commonly because patients are unable to take current medications because of their side effects, patients will need to learn how to move forward with HCV as part, but only part, of their lives. This "essential guide for the newly diagnosed" will be the foundation for the patient's understanding about how to live successfully and productively with HCV infection.

TERESA L. WRIGHT, M.D., is Chief of the Gastroenterology at the San Francisco Veterans Administration Medical Center and Professor of Medicine at the University of California, San Francisco. She has co-authored more than seventy original publications in peer-reviewed journals as well as more than twenty editorials and fifty chapters. The vast majority of these publications have been in the natural history of treatment of viral hepatitis C and B. She has been a visiting professor at sixteen universities in the U.S. and Canada. Dr. Wright is an associate editor of Hepatology, *has been on the editorial boards of* Gastroenterology, Antiviral Therapy, Gut *and the* American Journal of Medicine, *and is a member of the Council of the American Association for the the Study of Liver Diseases.*

Introduction

IF YOU'RE reading this book, chances are you or someone you love has just been diagnosed with hepatitis C (hep C).
Whether you feel shocked, frightened, angry, depressed, or
guilt-ridden, whether you're without signs of illness, or struggling with symptoms you can't ignore, this book is for you. It
will help you deal with every aspect of this chronic illness—a
potential time bomb that runs the gamut from extreme debili-
tation to no symptoms at all.

We have hepatitis C ourselves. Unfortunately, we learned
about it the hard way. When we met, we discovered that we
shared the same emotional needs, questions, and concerns, as do
many others who are infected. There was very little information
in 1990, when Lisa was diagnosed. When Cara was diagnosed in
2000, there were still no books that addressed the whole person
and met our emotional and social needs. We had to become
proactive—researching our illness and seeking support. We
wrote this book to help people like us—people infected with the
hepatitis C virus (HCV). We want you to know that you are not
alone.

For most of us, being diagnosed with hepatitis C is overwhelming. When we first wrote this book in 2001, hep C was called the "silent epidemic," due to lack of media attention and public awareness. Six years later, this disease is still surrounded in silence, ignorance and conflicting information. Some of us never hear of hep C until we're diagnosed, and when we tell our family and friends about our diagnosis, they have no idea what hep C is.

According to the Centers for Disease Control (CDC), hepatitis C is "the most common chronic blood-borne infection in the United States." The World Health Organization indicates that four million Americans or 1 in 50 have been infected. That's 1.8 percent of the U.S. population with approximately 36,000 new cases a year. An estimated 300 million people are infected worldwide.[1]

Following infection, there is:

○ An incubation period of two to 26 weeks, averaging six to seven weeks
○ A 75 to 85 percent chance of becoming chronically infected with the HCV virus. A disease is called "chronic" when it lasts for more than six months.
○ A 70 percent chance of developing chronic liver disease. Some people who carry the hep C virus don't have chronic inflammation of the liver.
○ A 10 to 20 percent chance of developing cirrhosis, usually over a period of 20 to 30 years.
○ A 1 to 5 percent chance of mortality from chronic liver disease. In the U.S., hep C kills 8,000 to 10,000 people each year.

This book is addressed to people who have just been diagnosed with hepatitis C. Seventy-five to 85 percent of those exposed to the virus develop chronic infection. But if you are chronically infected, there is an 80 to 90 percent chance that you will never develop cirrhosis, and an estimated 95 to 99 percent chance that you will not die from chronic liver disease.

While this data is reassuring, the uncertainties surrounding hep C can be incredibly frustrating. The HCV virus was only discovered in 1989, and still relatively little is known about its natural history, its full range of effects on the body, or the factors that determine whether or not an infected person will progress to end-stage liver disease. The information on these topics varies widely, and the first things we learn about HCV usually raise more questions than answers. So far there is no effective treatment for the majority of patients but volumes of advice on dietary changes and treatments that may potentially slow the progress of the disease.

This book offers an anchor in this sea of information and advice. Although it cannot answer the unknowns of hepatitis C, it provides a schedule that will help you take care of yourself emotionally, learn what you need to know about hepatitis C, and make the lifestyle changes you need to make at a pace that is right for you.

The good news is that hepatitis C is a "lazy" virus. It progresses slowly and often takes decades to affect people's health. Many people live for 30 or 40 years without experiencing symptoms, and there's a lot you can do to slow the progress of the virus and prevent liver damage. If you learn to take care of yourself, there's an excellent chance that you may never develop severe liver disease.

Nonetheless, it's ultimately up to you to manage your health care. Some of the most important steps you can take involve lifestyle changes, such as avoiding alcohol and drugs. For some of you this won't be a problem; for others, it will be the hardest part about having hep C. If this is an issue for you, once again, you are not alone. There are plenty of support groups and health care professionals who can help. But it's up to you to find them, consult them, and follow their guidance. Even the most skilled health care providers can do very little without your assistance.

This book will help you learn to take care of yourself. There's a lot you need to learn, but we've broken it down into chunks that are easy to absorb. We are no substitute for a medical doctor. Nonetheless, we do have something that most doctors won't have—the experience of living with hep C. Thus, we can help you learn to live with hepatitis C on a daily basis. For instance, we can assist you in dealing with the shock of being diagnosed and with some of the effects that hep C may have on your lifestyle and social life.

What happened to us

LISA MONTANARELLI: In June, 1990, when I was 22, I got sick with what seemed like the worst flu I'd ever had. I was so exhausted that I lay in bed for several weeks. I couldn't go near the kitchen, because the smell of food made me nauseous. I recovered slowly. At the time I never suspected I had hepatitis. Although I knew nothing about hep C, I knew that the generic symptoms of hepatitis were jaundice, dark urine, and light stools. I had none of these.

In September 1990, I got a letter from the Blood Bank saying that I had tested positive for hepatitis C, a virus that became chronic in 75 to 85 percent of the people who contracted it and could lead to severe liver disease. I was in grad school, so I saw a doctor at the university clinic. I think I was the first patient with hep C he'd ever seen. He explained that the "flu" I'd had in June was most likely a **seroconversion** illness, which means I got sick during the time that my body began producing **antibodies** to HCV. **Seroconversion** refers to the period between the initial exposure and the point at which laboratory tests indicate the presence of antibodies in the blood.

The doctor drew more blood, impressed me with the seriousness of the disease, and tried to help me figure out how I had gotten it. To this day I don't know exactly how I contracted hep C, but now I know that there are lots of ways I could have been exposed to the virus. I've had my ears pierced with needles that weren't properly sterilized; I've used other people's razors disinfected with rubbing alcohol; I've done lots of things that seem careless now that I know how hep C is transmitted. Like many people, I was operating under the assumption that hep C was like HIV, which dies quickly when exposed to air. Neither my doctor nor I could figure out how I'd contracted hep C. I'd always tried to look out for my health and safety— what had I done wrong? My doctor concluded—almost by default—that I'd gotten it sexually. Although hep C has a very low risk of sexual transmission, people weren't sure of that at the time. This left me even more confused, because I'd been practicing safer sex as well.

I was only 22 when I was diagnosed with hep C. I thought my life was over. I began researching immediately, but at the time little was known about the natural history of the disease. The virus had just been discovered in 1989—the previous year. Most doctors didn't know much about it. And when I told my friends I had hepatitis C, they invariably asked, "What's that?" A lot of people didn't take it very seriously because they'd never heard of hep C, and I didn't look ill. Fortunately, I haven't been ill with hepatitis for the last eleven years. Now doctors know that many people don't experience severe symptoms for two or three decades, and some never do. I believe I'm going to be healthy for a long time, but in 1990, that seemed very uncertain.

I've been very proactive about my health care from the beginning. I've talked to specialists and kept up on the latest research and treatments. Although I knew no one else with hep C in 1990, I learned a lot from watching friends with HIV deal with their illness and with the healthcare system. The first person I met with hep C—in 1991—was an AIDS activist named Richard, who was infected with both hep C and HIV and would eventually die of liver failure. He and others like him showed me that it was possible to live with chronic and terminal diseases that affected people's lives far more adversely than hep C has ever affected mine. I am particularly grateful for the work of ACT UP in the late 80s and the culture that emerged from it: as a result, people with all kinds of chronic conditions are more conscious and proactive regarding their health care.

In 1990 I knew no one else who had hep C. Most people didn't even know what it was. Around 1996 I began meeting a lot more people with HCV and talking to people who were recently diagnosed or undergoing treatment. When I told someone I had hep C, they often responded, "I know someone who has that!" In the last few years I've met more people than I can count. Every week I meet someone or hear of a friend of a friend who's been diagnosed. Many of them have had it for years without knowing it. After eleven years of living with hepatitis C, it's exciting to see this epidemic finally reaching public consciousness.

CARA BRUCE: In October 2000, about a month before my 27th birthday, I found out I had hepatitis C. I didn't know much about the disease, and as soon as my doctor told me, I felt as if I had been handed a death sentence. I was in shock. I didn't know how to deal with the fact that my lifespan might be greatly reduced. I called my parents immediately and cried my eyes out. They were scared as well.

We searched for information. Much of what I found on the Internet was wildly conflicting, and there weren't any books that addressed the specific lifestyle issues that I faced. I was 27 years old and single. How was I going to be able to take care of myself in the future? How could I change my lifestyle? Where could I go to meet people who didn't drink? Could I have sex again? I needed someone or something to help me deal with the confusion, depression, and pain of accepting the fact that I had a chronic illness and that I was going to have to change my life because of it.

As was true for Lisa, there were many ways I could have contracted the virus and to this day I am not sure how I got it. I was so sick that I couldn't get out of bed, and I threw up everything I ate. I was literally wasting away. At one point I weighed less than 100 pounds, and I looked like I was dying. I felt like I was dying. Through most of the writing of this book I have been recovering from an acute hepatitis sickness. Lisa helped me tremendously. Just knowing that she too had been through a serious illness and had gotten better gave me hope. I consider myself very lucky and value my life and my health more than I ever have before.

How we wrote this book together

A friend told Cara to call Lisa, who had had hepatitis C for 10 years. That phone call changed both our lives.

Lisa was at home in her San Francisco apartment when the phone rang. The voice on the other end was sobbing. Lisa asked her questions, gave her information, and helped her calm down. More than anything else, she related to Cara's story.

Although no two people are alike, Lisa had a fairly good idea what Cara was going through. She understood the shock of finding out in your twenties that you have a chronic illness. You'll never be in "perfect health," and in a sense, you've lost your youth, because you'll never be able to do some of the things that other young people take for granted. She also understood how isolated Cara must feel—being diagnosed with a disease that hardly anyone knows about.

When Cara started the conversation with Lisa, she was upset, but Lisa helped her. She explained that Cara wasn't going to die right away and that she was going to get better. She would start feeling better as she recovered from her **seroconversion** illness, although she had a high chance of developing chronic hep C. She related to everything that Cara was saying. Just hearing that someone had had the same symptoms and had gotten better was such a tremendous relief. And Lisa was living happily and had a great life. They immediately felt close. They discussed the fact that there was so much conflicting information and that there were very few books about hep C on the shelves, while there were tons of books on cancer and HIV. Cara was shocked at all of the information that Lisa was telling her—that there was this easily transmissible blood-borne illness, it was a major epidemic, and hardly anyone knew about it. She was outraged. She asked Lisa if she had ever thought of writing something about it and then suggested that they write something together.

Within a few weeks we had started discussing writing a book—one that answered all of the questions that we both had. Cara didn't know how she was going to go out and have a social life. She wasn't sure that anyone would ever fall in love with her and want to be with her, or if she could have sex. Lisa had had many of the same fears and uncertainties. It was important to both of us that the book we started to work on covered the emotional, mental, spiritual, and physical aspects of being diagnosed with a chronic illness. We wanted it to be for people like us—people with suddenly uncertain futures. We wanted to reassure people like you, who have just received your diagnosis, that many of your fears may be unfounded. There's a good chance that you can live a healthy life. Even people with severe liver damage have been able to improve their health and feel better. Unfortunately many people don't realize this and only think of the stigma that is attached to hep C. We have had problems with relationships and even friendships because of it. At the same time, we have many friends who are infected. We have both found that when we come out about having the virus, many people share their stories with us. The number of people we know who are infected is both staggering and depressing. But at the same time, we are all learning to live with it together.

Both of us were lucky enough to have a seroconversion illness. We say lucky because it alerted us to the fact that something was wrong. Many people with hep C don't know and inadvertently harm themselves through drinking and other behaviors, which healthier livers can handle. We hope you will never experience the symptoms of severe liver disease. In this book we suggest ways to live that may help you stay healthier longer. Living with hepatitis C is a constant balancing act. The key is to avoid substances that can harm your liver, without sacrificing your quality of life. Before you were diagnosed with hep C, you most likely didn't spend much time thinking about how to keep your liver healthy. It takes time to adjust to this way of thinking, but it will get easier. We hope our book makes it easier for you.

How to use this book

We wrote this book for people who have just been diagnosed with hep C. Most of us are overwhelmed with the shock of diagnosis. We're also overwhelmed with the amount of information we have to learn and the changes we have to make in our lifestyles. The good news is that you don't have to do everything at once. This book will make the process easier for you. We have organized the information in short chapters, which you can absorb quickly and easily. You will learn how to live with hep C step-by-step and one day at a time.

The first chapter, Day 1, deals with what you may be feeling on the day you receive your diagnosis. It's OK if you don't start the book on the day you're diagnosed. We still suggest you start at the beginning, because the feelings you experience on the day you're diagnosed won't go away immediately after the first day.

The book gives you a schedule for learning what you need to know about hep C and making the necessary changes. We encourage you to adapt the schedule to your needs and read the book at your own pace. The book guides you through your first year of living with hepatitis C, starting with the day you're diagnosed. The first seven chapters are designed for you to read each day of the first week. The next three chapters guide you through the second, third, and fourth weeks of the first month, and the next eleven chapters provide a program for learning about hep C and taking care of yourself during the remaining months of the first year.

Each chapter is divided into two sections, called "Living" and "Learning." The purpose of this division is to strike a balance between addressing the emotional and social issues you may face in your day-to-day life ("Living") and providing facts about hep C and information you need to manage your health ("Learning"). Terms in **boldface** are defined in the glossary, at the end of the book.

We also designed this book to be interactive. It's filled with exercises and questions to help you identify your needs and feelings, as well as practical questions, such as those you need to ask your doctor. It's important to keep a journal in which you record your answers and write down anything else that comes up for you. This will allow you to look back and recognize what you are experiencing and how far you have come.

We will not prescribe

We are not medical doctors, and we will not prescribe for you. We do not tell you which treatments we think are best. Research findings on hepatitis C change rapidly. Treatments that seem most effective today will undoubtedly be outdated in the next few years.

Instead of recommending any specific treatments, we describe a variety of options. Week 4 focuses on conventional treatments while Month 2 gives an overview of complementary and alternative treatments. Our aim is to provide background information, so that you can understand new treatments as they come along and work with your doctor to find a plan that works for you. In Month 7 we provide a chapter on keeping up-to-date and doing research that will give you tools to find the most current information.

Nothing we say can substitute for a doctor's advice. Although we tell you which vitamins, supplements, and herbs are toxic to the liver and which are liver friendly, we urge you to consult your doctor or herbalist before you embark on any vitamin or herbal regimen. We also urge you to check with your doctor before you start a new diet or exercise plan or before you stop or start taking any pharmaceutical or recreational drug.

Where our focus is

Since we begin with the day you're diagnosed, the first few chapters focus on the shock of diagnosis and what you need to do right away. We also concentrate on the most urgent questions you may have, such as:

- ○ Am I going to die? How much time do I have left?
- ○ Is there a cure?
- ○ What can I do to stay as healthy as possible?
- ○ What did I do to get this?
- ○ How do I avoid giving it to other people?
- ○ Can I still have sex?
- ○ Am I going to be sick for the rest of my life?
- ○ Do I have to give up my dreams and goals?
- ○ How do I change my social life?

Hopefully our answers to these questions will allay some of your worst fears.

This book also focuses on how you can prevent liver damage. Although we provide overviews of a variety of treatments you need to know about—including **interferon** and **liver transplants**, neither of us can speak first-hand about being treated with interferon, or having a liver transplant. We have, however, included personal stories of people who can. Fortunately, most of you will not be receiving treatment or transplants during your first year after diagnosis. The section on transplants is meant to inform you of the issues surrounding organ donation and how they are relevant to your life. It is not meant to prepare you to receive a transplant.

Although both of us have had bouts of acute hepatitis in the form of sero-conversion illnesses, we cannot speak firsthand about living with severe liver disease either. Many people get tested and diagnosed only after they experience severe symptoms, but whether you have symptoms or not, we hope this book will help you improve your quality of life and stay as healthy as you can for as long as possible.

When we talk with other people with hep C, we often find that we have similar issues and concerns. We have tried to address the issues that are most common. Nonetheless, no two people with hep C are alike, and some sections of this book may not be relevant to you. For instance, we have included sections on avoiding drugs and alcohol, having kids, and **coinfection** with HIV. If these topics are not an issue for you, feel free to skip them.

In writing this book, we have also tried to address issues that other books don't cover. Unlike most other books on hepatitis C, we give specific guidelines on how to prevent hep C transmission through drug paraphernalia. For those of you who have never used drugs or don't use them currently, these sections won't be relevant. Nonetheless, we included this material because, according to the World Health Organization (WHO), 90 percent of the people infected in developed nations contracted HCV through IV drug use or receiving contaminated blood products. The CDC says that sharing needles and other "works" accounts for 60 to 80 percent of HCV transmission in the United States.[2] The National Institute of Drug Abuse (NIDA) says hepatitis C infection happens soon after people start using IV drugs. Fifty to 80 percent are infected within six to 12 months, and as many as 95 percent contract HCV after five years of using. Relatively little is being done to educate people about how to prevent this route of transmission. But lack of information is not an effective strategy for preventing the transmission of hep C. However you got this disease, your health matters, and you deserve accurate information on how to keep yourself as safe and healthy as possible.

While we address the issue of IV drug use, we also try to dispel the myth that this is "the main route of transmission" throughout the world. From a global perspective, the use of nonsterilized medical equipment is by far the most common means of transmission. Although IV drug use is a global problem, it accounts for only a small proportion of HCV infections world-wide. It is only a significant means of transmission in industrialized nations, where medical procedures are usually performed with sterilized instruments under sterile conditions.

Unlike other books, we also talk about sex and dating with hep C. These are very real issues for people living with a stigmatized infectious disease. Again, we cannot tell you exactly how to solve these problems, but we offer ways to make things easier.

Keep on learning

By the end of your first year with hepatitis C, we hope that you will want to continue your learning process and share your knowledge with others. Hep C is called the "silent epidemic." The more educated we are as patients, and the more we can educate others, the faster we will break this silence and destroy some of the damaging stigmas facing people with hep C. We also hope that you will be better able to discern accurate information from all the hype in the media.

New information is constantly appearing on the Internet and news articles are coming out more and more frequently. We help you find these resources in Month 7. And we list resources at the end of most chapters. Finally, in the resource section we list Web sites and organizations that can help you stay up-to-date with the newest treatments and discoveries about hepatitis C.

Hepatitis C is a chronic illness. There is no effective treatment for the majority of patients. While that sounds bleak, the good news is that it is a manageable disease, and it is possible to live a healthy and happy life. With proper knowledge and care, most people will live without symptoms or problems for many years. Being diagnosed with a chronic illness has sometimes been called a "blessing in disguise." It forces you to take care of yourself and become more aware of changes in your body and your life. It certainly has been this way for us. Hep C has taught us to change our lifestyles, diets, and exercise habits. It has helped us make better choices in our lives and realize what is truly important to us. These are lessons we are glad to have learned early, and we feel our lives will be better because of them. We actually feel healthier and more energetic than ever before.

Of course, having hepatitis C does not always bring boundless joy. There are many problems that you will continually face. Some of us will experience more detrimental side effects and symptoms, and some of us will be stigmatized and possibly ostracized. We are sorry about your diagnosis, but we do want you to know that you are not alone. An estimated 300 million people worldwide have been exposed to hepatitis C. Many experts believe this estimate may be low. As public awareness increases and people get tested, that number will grow. Chances are you already know someone with hep C, someone who understands and knows what you are going through. In the resource section and in the section called "Building a Support System" in Week 3, we list ways to find some of these people. You are not alone.

So You Have Hep C. What Now?

This is not a death sentence

"For the last year I'd been feeling so tired I couldn't get out of bed. It took a few doctors to figure out what was wrong with me. When I got the diagnosis, I thought I was going to die right there in the doctor's office. I'd always thought of myself as a healthy person. I spent the first day in a daze, not knowing what to do."

—CHRIS D.

"My husband just got diagnosed with hep C. He doesn't want to talk about it. I'm so scared. What comes next?"

—ELISA S.

IF YOU'RE like most of us, your diagnosis came as a shock. Being told you have a chronic illness can be incredibly frightening. You may feel helpless, overwhelmed, and out-of-control, especially if you're experiencing symptoms. Your fears are real and valid, but hepatitis C is not a death sentence. Most of us will outlive our disease and die from unrelated causes.

You are not helpless. The one thing you can control is your ability to take charge of your health and get your needs met. No matter what stage of the disease you're in, you're fortunate to have been diagnosed. The simple fact that you know you have hep C puts you in a position of power, because there are plenty of things you can do to take care of yourself and reduce your risk of future illness. Hepatitis C is a manageable illness, and it is entirely possible to live a rich, full, healthy life. In fact, many of us live healthier lives after we're diagnosed with hepatitis C.

Throughout the following chapters, we will be discussing the first steps you can take to live a healthy life with hep C. But first you may need to deal with the shock of diagnosis and the feelings that emerge during the first week. Some common reactions include:

○ Fear: "What's going to happen to me?"
○ Anger: "Why did this have to happen to me? It's so unfair!"
○ Sadness: "It ruined my life."
○ Guilt: "Why did I ever do this to myself?"
○ Confusion: "What do I do now?"

It's unlikely that you'll experience all these emotions on the first day. You may be completely calm right now. But all of these feelings are bound to come up during your first year of living with hepatitis C. Whatever you're going through, this book will help you develop a practice for dealing with these emotions as they arise.

"I got hepatitis C giving birth to my daughter. I had to have a cesarean section, and they gave me blood. I found out about my hep years later, when I was constantly tired. The biggest surprise was that there was nothing they could do. I had such an overwhelming feeling of hopelessness and confusion. And also anger. How could this have happened? How could I have gotten a virus in a hospital?"

—NANCY M.

"I used IV drugs once or twice years ago, back when I used to party. The other day I found out I have hep C. I could just kill myself. I hate myself for having fucked around like that. I would do anything to take it all back."

—MARK G.

Focus on the present, not on how you got hep C

Your first reactions to your diagnosis may depend a lot on how you contracted the virus. Many of us may have no idea how or when we were infected. The news most likely came as a shock. If you received contaminated blood products, you're most likely angry: "Why did this have to happen to me?" If you got hep C from sharing IV needles, you may have to deal with guilt: "Why did I do this to myself?" Your biggest challenge might be to forgive yourself.

"I have both HIV and hep C. For the first two years after I found out, I thought I knew exactly who had infected me with both, and I obsessed about it. Or rather, I obsessed about that person. It was really unhealthy and counterproductive. I don't really know how I got infected or when. I was just looking for a scapegoat—a way of saying, 'It's not my fault.' What I really needed was to forgive myself."

—KEVIN T.

"In one hep C support group I went to, the room was divided between people who had gotten hep C from sharing IV needles and people who had gotten it from blood transfusions or some other means. Some of the people who'd never used IV drugs thought that they didn't deserve hep C, and the IV drug users did. I kept telling them to focus on the present, not on how they got the illness or whether they deserved it or not."

—JIM C.

Not all hep C support groups are like this. Unfortunately you may run into some people who treat you as if you deserved hep C. We want you to know that, however you got this disease, you don't deserve it. Hep C is not a punishment, and at this point, it isn't productive to dwell on what you could have done to avoid getting hep C. Some of you may also be angry about receiving contaminated blood products. In either case, the best suggestion we can offer is to focus on the present. Don't ask what you could have done differently. Ask what you can do now. This book will help you answer that question for yourself.

You may go through the "five stages of grief"

It's important to give yourself time to accept your diagnosis and to grieve. As your experience of living with hep C unfolds, you'll find yourself going through layers of feelings and stages of acceptance. Many of us experience the "five stages of grief." These include:

1. Denial and Isolation
2. Anger
3. Bargaining
4. Depression
5. Acceptance[1]

These "stages" represent some of the feelings and coping mechanisms we go through in the process of accepting any unwanted change—whether we're mourning the loss of our job, the loss of our health, or facing our own mortality. Professionals who deal with grief know that the process is far more complicated: we can go through these stages repeatedly in any order, and often the stages coexist side by side. Yes, we can be angry, depressed, and in denial all at the same time. There's no standard way of dealing with loss. Each of us goes through our own process at our own pace. The important thing is that you do deal with your emotions. Writing down what you are experiencing is one way to ensure that you don't simply repress them so that you don't have to feel them. They will only come back. Once you have accepted that you have hep C and have accepted how you got it (if you know), you will be ready to live comfortably in the present with your disease.

Many of us have to face depression. In fact, some people report depression as a symptom of hep C. It is common to feel sad right after your diagnosis, but if you are experiencing signs of depression months later, you may want to find a support group or talk to a therapist. We discuss ways of dealing with depression in Week 3 and provide guidelines for choosing a therapist in Month 8.

Once you take control of your life with hep C, you will begin to feel better. Managing your life with hep C means everything from changing your drinking or drug habits to eating well, exercising, and taking herbs. How you live your life is ultimately up to you, but whatever you decide, you'll feel much better with more knowledge and more choices.

Putting things in perspective

> *"Having hep C is a blessing in disguise. Now I enjoy every moment. I really do stop to smell the flowers. It taught me how to make the most of my life now."*
>
> —JACKIE T.

In order to accept your hep C status, you have to look at hep C in relation to the rest of your life. This may be a good time to remind yourself of the positive things. As we said above, you may feel out of control. But hep C is a lot more manageable than many other aspects of your life. For instance, you can't control your past or other people's reactions, but you have the power to take care of your health and your body.

Hepatitis C can give us a different perspective. We live in a goal-oriented society, and many of us never enjoy the present because we spend most of our time working toward our future goals. Since none of us knows how long we'll be around, it's important not to put our dreams on hold.

But it's equally important not to throw our lives away. Hepatitis C reminds us to live in the present—but carefully. If we take care of ourselves in the present, we have a much better chance of a healthy future. You'll realize that living with hep C or any chronic illness is a daily balancing act, in which you'll constantly be weighing your present quality of life against your future health. Do you want to enjoy an occasional glass of wine at dinner, or abstain completely in order to tax your liver as little as possible? If you're like most of us, you haven't spent much time thinking about your liver's health. As we said in our introduction, it takes time to adjust to this way of thinking. It may feel tedious and frustrating at first. But it will become second nature and help you make decisions in every aspect of your life.

Having hepatitis C has affected both our lives in drastic ways. For Cara, having hep C has forced her to come to terms with herself. It has made her value her future, rethink her priorities, and focus on the present. Lisa can hardly imagine her life without hep C. She's had it since 1990 and she would be so different if she hadn't gotten it. It made her think about what she wanted. She is happy with her life now, and she wouldn't have it any other way.

"When I have a big decision to make, I ask myself: 'What would I do if I knew I was going to die tomorrow?' and 'What would I do if I knew I was going to live to be a hundred?'"

—GEORGE C.

"I used to do whitewater kayaking and all kinds of high-risk sports that could have killed me really easily, but none of it ever got to me as much as the day-to-day uncertainty of living with hep C. There's just no end to it."

—FRANK MILES

"I'm a teacher at a school, and we had a blood drive. I gave blood and was shocked when the letter came back saying that I had hepatitis C. I went to my doctor and found out that I had hepatitis C. I had never heard of it and was devastated. It was the biggest shock of my life."

—TIM K.

Start keeping a journal

Start a journal devoted to your emotional and physical well-being. During the first few weeks following your diagnosis, use your journal to record your feelings as they come up and figure out what you need to do to take care of yourself at that time. Try to write in it each day—even if you just jot down how you're feeling. This journal will help you see what's working, as you begin making changes in your diet, exercise, and lifestyle. It will also help you keep track of your progress if you pursue treatment.

IN A SENTENCE:

> *The first step toward living with hepatitis C is accepting that you have it*

learning

What Is Hepatitis?
What Is Hep C?

"Hepatitis" means inflammation of the liver

THERE ARE a number of possible causes of hepatitis:

○ Too much of a substance that is toxic to the liver, such as large quantities of alcohol, or Tylenol.
○ The immune system attacking part of the body. This is called **autoimmune hepatitis**.
○ A viral agent. Viral agents that cause hepatitis are designated by letters: hepatitis A (HAV), hep B (HBV), hep C (HCV), and the less common D, E, and G.

Hepatitis A through E designate a variety of viruses that attack the liver. Hepatitis A was discovered in 1973 and hepatitis B was discovered in 1965. Hepatitis A is primarily fecal to oral, although it is usually transmitted through an indirect route, such as a contaminated water supply or contaminated tableware. HAV is an acute illness that is not chronic. Most people recover completely with lifelong immunity to HAV infection.

Hepatitis B is passed blood-to-blood and through sexual intercourse. Before the virus was discovered, some people contracted HBV through blood products. Nowadays blood is screened for HBV, and it is most often transmitted through IV drug use, unprotected sex, or from mother to child. There's a widespread myth that all types of hepatitis are sexually transmitted, but actually hepatitis B is the only one that is easily spread through sexual contact. Some people become carriers or develop chronic hepatitis, but 90 to 95 percent of adults infected with HBV clear the virus and acquire lifelong immunity.

What hepatitis A and B have in common:

○ They are rarely chronic
○ Both cause acute protracted flulike illness and sometimes jaundice, the yellowing of the skin and eyes
○ Both can be prevented through vaccine.

If you've had hep A or B in the past, you probably have **antibodies**. Antibodies are proteins that fight infections. Antibodies fit into molecules called **antigens** on the surface of the virus the way a key fits into a lock. Once antibodies attach to the virus's surface, the body's white blood cells can locate the virus and fight the infection. In most cases of hep A, hep B, and many other viral infections, your body's immune system succeeds in fighting off the virus, and after the virus is eradicated, you still have antibodies, which protect you from getting the same virus again in the future. Hep C is different. Only 15 to 25 percent of people infected with hep C "clear" the virus and have antibodies but no detectable virus in their blood. The other 75 to 85 percent become chronically infected: Their immune systems don't succeed in eliminating the hep C virus, so they still have the virus as well as antibodies.

Not much is known about hepatitis D and E. These viruses are less common than A, B, and C, and some of them may even be variants of A, B, and C. Hepatitis D only occurs in people who have hepatitis B. A person with an HBV/HDV coinfection may have more severe acute disease and a higher risk of fulminant hepatitis compared with those infected with HBV alone. Since hepatitis D only occurs with hepatitis B, the vaccine for B will also work for D. However, there is no way to prevent an HDV superinfection once a person has HBV. E has the same symptoms as A, but usually occurs in Mexico, Central America, and India. There is no vaccine for hepatitis E. Several years ago, scientists identified another virus, which they called hepatitis G or GBV, but this virus does not seem to cause significant liver damage. Hepatitis E is extremely rare and usually occurs in places with inadequate sanitation. As with hepatitis A it is passed fecal to oral, most often in polluted drinking water. Travelers to endemic areas should be aware. Hepatitis G lives in the blood without causing any apparent illness. It does not appear to be infectious, yet 900 to 2,000 cases of HGV are discovered each year in the United States.

What is hepatitis C?

I had hepatitis back in the 70s. I thought I'd gotten over it. No one told me it was chronic. I don't think they knew back then. So I just went about my regular business for 25 years—not knowing I had to take any precautions. A couple of months ago I found out I have hep C and I'm at stage 1 fibrosis. I'm really lucky, considering I've had it for 25 years.

— HANNAH D.

In 1989 researchers discovered that a condition known as non-A-non-B hepatitis was actually caused by a viral agent. They named it hepatitis C.

The virus was not discovered earlier due to its unusually small size. Nonetheless, analysis of blood products from the 1940s and 50s shows that the HCV virus has been around for at least 50 years. Peter Simmonds, Ph.D., a virologist from the University of Edinburgh, speculates that hep C has been in the human population for several centuries. The virus may have been confined to a small region of Southeast Asia, until the twentieth century, when people began migrating in and out of that area. Population upheavals and new medical technology, such as blood transfusions, allowed the virus to contaminate the worldwide blood supply and spread throughout the world. Experts believe that HCV reached epidemic proportions in the post–World War II era. Blood samples from the postwar era show that the virus spread through blood transfusions, through the use of nonsterilized equipment in mass inoculation programs, and through medicines containing blood products, which scientists began to manufacture in the 1960s. Finally, the popularization of IV drug use helped the epidemic spread through industrialized nations, where sterilization of medical equipment is a more common practice.[3]

According to the Centers for Disease Control (CDC), hepatitis C is the most common chronic blood-borne infection in the United States. The World Health Organization indicates that four million Americans or 1 in 50 have been infected. That's 1.8 percent of the U.S. population with approximately 36,000 new cases a year. An estimated 300 million people are infected worldwide.

Following infection, there is:

○ An incubation period of two to 26 weeks, averaging six to seven weeks
○ A 75 to 85 percent chance of becoming chronically infected with the HCV virus. A disease is called "chronic" when it lasts for more than six months.
○ A 70 percent chance of developing chronic liver disease. Some people who carry the hep C virus don't have chronic inflammation of the liver.
○ A 10 to 20 percent chance of developing cirrhosis, usually over a period of 20 to 30 years.
○ A 1 to 5 percent chance of mortality from chronic liver disease. In the United States, hep C kills 8,000 to 10,000 people each year.

The numbers of those infected are staggering: over 300 million worldwide, or 5 percent of the global population. In the U.S. alone, four million or 1.8 percent are HCV positive. Most of these people don't know they have it, since as many as 80 percent of those infected can show no symptoms for 20 years or more. Nonetheless, the virus can ravage the liver, even when there are no signs of illness. Hepatitis C now ranks as the number one cause of death from liver disease, and death rates are expected to triple over the next 10 to 20 years.

My grandmother died of cirrhosis. She got hep C through a blood transfusion back in the 50s.

—PEGGY J.

What is a virus?

A **virus** is made of genetic instructions (**DNA** or **RNA**), encased in a capsule, or "**capsid**." Unlike cells and bacteria, viruses aren't really alive, because they can't carry out the chemical reactions they need to grow and reproduce on their own. Viruses act like living organisms in that they replicate their own genetic instructions and pass these instructions on to their offspring: They make copies of themselves—individual virus particles called virions. But viruses can't replicate on their own: They need to occupy the cells of a living organism (you) and use the cells' enzymes to make new virions. The hep C virus is a parasite, and your cells are the hosts that the virus needs to replicate itself. HCV is considered a very "successful" virus in the sense that it rarely kills its host: 95 percent of people infected die from unrelated causes.

Hepatitis C is a single-stranded RNA virus of the Flaviviridae family. It is not related to hepatitis A or B, but to the viruses that cause yellow fever, Japanese encephalitis, and bovine diarrhea.

The hep C virus mainly infects liver cells. It enters the cell through a receptor complex by a mechanism that is not fully understood. In the **cytoplasm**, the solution surrounding the nucleus of the cell, HCV sheds its envelope and releases its single-strand genome. The virus then starts using the host cell to reproduce itself. It takes over the host cell's enzymes and forces the host cell to follow the virus's genetic instructions and make new virus particles. We discuss this process in more detail in the section called "Trends in Research and Development" in Month 3. Unlike the **Human Immunodeficiency Virus** (HIV), hep C is not a retrovirus. HIV enters the nucleus of the host cell and integrates its own genetic instructions into the cell's DNA, so that when the cell reproduces it passes the virus's genetic instructions onto its offspring, which become factories for making new viruses. In contrast, the hep C virus never enters the host cell's nucleus, but lives in the cytoplasm, the solution inside the cell surrounding the nucleus. Theoretically, the fact that hep C doesn't integrate itself into the host cell's DNA should make the HCV virus easier to eradicate. But as we discuss later, the current standard treatment, a combination of pegylated interferon and ribavirin, does not get rid of the virus in nearly 50 percent of patients.

Viruses replicate differently, depending on whether they are made of **DNA (deoxyribonucleic acid)**, the double-stranded genetic instructions, or **RNA (ribonucleic acid)**, the single-stranded genetic instructions. When DNA viruses replicate, they have a quality-control mechanism that makes sure that the new virus has exactly the same DNA as the parent virus. RNA viruses don't have this quality-control mechanism: This means they have no way of making sure that the new virus has the same DNA as the parent. They thus have a much higher rate of mutation. **Mutations** are small changes in genetic material.

Hep C is an RNA virus. This means it mutates rapidly. Just think of millions of tiny virions constantly replicating and producing new genetic variations of the virus. Some of these mutations will be more resistant to drugs than others. This is why hep C is so difficult to treat with antiviral therapy. New genetic variations of hep C are constantly being produced in each of our bodies. Although there are infinitely many variations of hep C, six basic **genotypes**, or genetic variations, and 50 subtypes have been identified.[4] Some strains of hep C are so distinct that some scientists think they are actually different viruses.

HCV genotypes are classified according to the part of the world where they most commonly occur:

○ Genotype 1a is mostly found in North and South America and Australia.
○ Genotype 1b is prevalent in North America, Europe and Japan.
○ Genotype 2a is mainly found in China and Japan.
○ Genotype 2b is the most common subtype of 2 in the United States and Northern Europe. It also occurs in Japan, Taiwan, and China.
○ Genotype 2c is the subtype of 2 most common in Western and Southern Europe.
○ Genotype 3 is common in Scotland and throughout the UK, Europe and to a lesser extent in the United States.
○ Genotype 3a predominates in Australia and southern Asia.
○ Genotype 4 is prevalent in the Middle East and in Northern and Central Africa.
○ Genotype 4a is most common is Egypt. There is a high incidence of 4c in Central Africa.

○ Genotype 5a is mostly confined to South Africa.

○ Genotype 6 occurs mainly in Asia, particularly Hong Kong. Genotype 6a is restricted to Hong Kong, Macau, and Vietnam.[5]

The type most common in North America is called 1a, and the most common in Europe is 1b. Types 4 through 6 are very rare in the United States.

HCV primarily congregates in the liver. Scientists believe it damages the liver in two ways: The virus directly invades liver cells; it also triggers an **autoimmune** response, in which the body's immune system attacks liver cells, mistaking them for viruses, bacteria, or some other foreign invader. When the body is infected, the immune system reacts to the invader by producing white blood cells and **antibodies**. This immune response to the virus leads to chronic liver disease. The chronic inflammation leads to the formation of scar tissue in the liver—a process called **fibrosis**. This scar tissue replaces healthy liver tissue, and as normal liver function decreases, problems arise. These can include **coagulopathy**, disturbances in blood clotting that can make people bruise easily and bleed profusely from minor cuts, and **jaundice**, yellowing of skin and eyes due to inadequate processing of **bilirubin**. We elaborate on coagulopathy in the chapter on the stages of liver disease in Month 7, and we define bilirubin in Day 4, "Symptoms You Might Be Experiencing."

The HCV virus is extremely virulent, which means that small amounts of virus can cause intense illness. Nonetheless, the quantity of virus in the blood, called the **viral load**, does not seem to correspond to the degree of illness. Many people with high viral loads experience no symptoms and have little or no liver damage. At this point, scientists don't really know how or if genotype and viral load correspond to the progression of disease.

Unfortunately, HCV is extremely infectious—you can get it through a single exposure to a very small quantity of virus. It is also resilient—meaning it is hard to get rid of. Even when it seems as if all virus has been eliminated from the host's body, it can still reappear. This is incredibly frustrating for patients and doctors researching drug therapy. In some cases, it seems as if the person has been "cured" because his or her viral load disappears. But the virus can come back two or three years later.

*"I went in to get an HIV test. I'd prepared myself to find out
I had HIV. I knew what I'd do if I tested positive.
I knew what my next step would be. When I went back to get
my test results, they told me I didn't have HIV. I was relieved.
But then they told me I had this other thing called hep C.
I hadn't even heard of that. At first I wished I had tested
positive for HIV instead of hep C. Now I understand that
was foolish. At the time, I was thinking that there had been
all this research on HIV. Why did I have to get something
that was untreatable and that they knew so much less about?"*

—FRANK MILES

IN A SENTENCE:

> *Hepatitis C is a viral form of hepatitis, meaning "inflammation of
> the liver."*

DAY 2

living

What You Need
to Do Right Away

*"In 1997 I was getting so sick that I had to stop
working. None of the doctors I went to could tell
what was wrong with me, until somebody tested
my liver enzymes, and they were really high. I got
tested for hep C and tested positive. The doctor
told me it was a terminal disease, which isn't true.
But I was so scared that I stopped drinking
immediately. I had been a heavy drinker, and I
have not had a drop of alcohol since."*

—PAULINE M.

IN THE previous chapter we described living with hep C
as a balancing act, challenging us to weigh what we want to
do in the present against our future health. Although you may
feel out of control and profoundly unbalanced after receiving
your diagnosis, there are things you can do right away to take
care of your liver and improve your health and general sense
of well being.

16

○ Get vaccinated for hepatitis A and B.

○ If you drink, stop as much as you can.

○ If you use drugs, stop as much as you can.

○ If you use IV drugs, be sure not to share or reuse works.

○ Stop taking medications and herbs that are toxic to your liver. See list in Day 7. Ask your doctor about Tylenol. It may be damaging to your liver in doses of more than 2g per day, or when taken with alcohol.

○ Quit smoking.

○ If you believe that you have been infected with HCV in the last several months, consult a specialist about your treatment options as soon as possible. A recent study found that early treatment may prevent hep C from becoming chronic.[1]

Many of us find it is hardest to make lifestyle changes, which can include anything from altering your diet to quitting an addiction. Some of us hardly need to modify our lives at all. Others face decisions that seem next to impossible. This is no cause for alarm. These things take time. If you are dependent on alcohol, drugs, or nicotine, you know that you didn't acquire these addictions in one day. No one expects you to get rid of them in one day either. Everything starts with the first step. In Week 2 we will help you decide what modifications you need to make and how to prioritize them and come up with a schedule for transforming your lifestyle. The key to living a healthy life with hep C is learning to *live with* your hep C. The disease takes so long to progress that most of us have lots of time to modify our lifestyles. Nonetheless, we recommend that you begin as soon as possible. Hep C can be a valuable teacher, helping us make positive changes in our lives.

Get vaccinated!

The easiest thing on your to-do list is getting vaccinated for hepatitis A and hepatitis B. Even if you usually avoid conventional western medicine, it's crucial that you get these **vaccines**. You can get them at your doctor's office or local health clinic—but get them as soon as you can, because hep A or B can be fatal on top of hep C. If you've had hep A or B in the past, you most likely have antibodies. But ask for a test just to make sure. A positive result means you're already immune. A negative test result means you need to get immunized. The hep A vaccine requires two shots over a six-month period, while hep B is three shots over six months. The combination vaccine for hep A and B also requires three shots over six months. These vaccines work by injecting dead viruses into your bloodstream. Your body will mount an immune reaction and produce antibodies to the viruses, but you will not contract the disease.

After your hep B vaccinations, it's important to get tested again, since not everyone becomes immune after the first series of injections. Older people, overweight people, and smokers are less likely to become immune after the initial series.

Alcohol: Enemy number 1

If you have hep C, one of the key things you can do to protect your liver is to stop or cut back on your alcohol consumption. Heavy drinking seems to be one of the major factors contributing to the development of cirrhosis in patients with hep C. Ethanol, the type of alcohol in drinks, is extremely toxic. Because it is soluble in both water and fat, it can enter and damage any organ in the body. The liver is responsible for protecting the body (and itself) from alcohol by breaking it down into less toxic byproducts. After an enzyme called alcohol dehydrogenase converts ethanol into an even more poisonous byproduct, acetaldehyde, another liver enzyme, aldehyde dehydrogenase, converts acetaldehyde into water, carbon dioxide, and acetate (a kind of vinegar that is harmless to the body). This is how the liver metabolizes most of the alcohol we drink. The liver can also break down alcohol through a different method known as the microsomal ethanol oxidizing system (MEOS). When a person drinks excessively, these mechanisms get overwhelmed and can't break down alcohol fast enough—allowing alcohol to damage the liver and other organs.

There is conflicting evidence regarding alcohol's role in increasing the risk of cirrhosis in hep C patients.[2] For instance, a team of NIH-supported researchers showed that alcohol increases the replication of the HCV virus in human liver cell lines grown in the laboratory.[3]

According to the 2002 United States National Institutes of Health (NIH) Consensus Statement, 30 grams of alcohol (three drinks) a day for men and 20 grams (two drinks) a day for women increases the risk of liver damage associated with hep C. The CDC says that even moderate drinking (more than 10 grams or one drink per day) may accelerate liver damage in hep C patients.[4]

It is not known whether light drinking increases HCV-related fibrosis, but no studies have demonstrated that any alcohol is "safe" for people with hep C. Since light alcohol consumption has cardiovascular benefits, middle-aged men and others who are at risk for cardiovascular disease might ask their doctors if the benefits of very light drinking outweigh the risks.

For alcoholics or people who find it difficult to cut back on drinking, Week 2 provides guidelines for getting sober or greatly reducing your intake. Be sure to consult your doctor and seek the support of a **detox** or 12-step program. If you use both alcohol and drugs and can't give up both right away, you can start by quitting one or the other. This is a method of harm reduction, which is not as liver-friendly as staying clean and sober, but it is something you can do immediately to stay as safe and healthy as possible. Harm reduction has saved many people's lives.

Some of us like to have an occasional drink. This is a quality-of-life choice, and it is a good example of the balancing act we discussed in Day 1. If your liver is relatively healthy, one glass of wine won't do much damage. Nonetheless, many people with hep C have a hard time tolerating alcohol. It also compromises the immune system, so the virus can multiply unchecked.

Some recreational drugs can be toxic to your liver

Your liver processes almost everything you take in through your mouth, lungs, and skin. What you put into your body is ultimately your own decision, but we encourage you to educate yourself and make informed choices. Many recreational drugs are toxic to your liver and suppress your immune system, which is doubly dangerous to people with HCV. Even though some drugs are safer than others, they could be cut with anything. Sometimes the cut is more toxic than the drug. Living a "drug lifestyle," in which you don't eat, don't sleep, and stay up all night, can also damage your overall health and accelerate the progress of hepatitis C. In Week 2 we go into detail about prioritizing lifestyle changes. We discuss specific drugs and how they affect the liver in the Learning section of Day 7.

Some pharmaceuticals can also be toxic to your liver

The fact that a drug is legal doesn't mean it's safe. Many pharmaceuticals can be toxic to your liver—especially when taken in large doses or in combination. Be sure to consult a hep C–aware doctor about any medications you're taking. Here's a list of medications that can be toxic to your liver.

O Steroid hormones
O Acetaminophen (Tylenol)/paracetamol. Ask your doctor about Tylenol. It may be damaging to your liver in doses of more than 2g per day, or when taken with alcohol.
O Birth control pills
O Aspirin and disprin are dangerous for those with severe liver damage.
O Ibuprofen
O Benzodiazepines, especially Halcion
O Barbituates
O Diazepam tranquilizers and sleeping pills
O Some antidepressants.

This list is not exhaustive and does not substitute for a doctor's advice. We go into this topic in more detail in Day 7.

IN A SENTENCE:

> *The first things you need to do are get vaccinated for hep A and B and quit or cut back on alcohol and other liver-toxic substances.*

learning

Transmission: How Did I Get This? How Can I Avoid Giving It to Other People?

HAVING HEP C doesn't mean you have to go into quarantine. You can't get hep C or give it to other people by hugging, kissing, or sharing the same glass. Hep C is a blood-borne virus, meaning it can only enter the bloodstream through any behavior or situation allowing blood-to-blood contact.

The most common means of transmission

○ The use of nonsterile medical equipment. According to the WHO, the major means of transmission in nonindustrialized nations are unsterilized injection equipment and unscreened blood products. This is the most common way hep C is spread worldwide. In developed nations, 90 percent of transmission occurs through IV drug use or receiving contaminated blood products.

○ Receiving contaminated blood products. In the United States 25 percent contracted the virus through contaminated blood products. The first reliable blood-screening test was developed in 1992. This means that anyone who received a blood transfusion or blood clotting factors before 1992 is at risk. Now the risk of contracting hepatitis C from a blood product is 1 in 1 million or less than 1 in 2 million units of blood.

○ Sharing IV needles or other **"works,"** including cookers, cotton, spoons, water, ties, and anything else that could have blood in or on it. Seventy-nine percent of IV drug users have hep C. Thirty percent of these people only used IV drugs once or occasionally.

MANY PEOPLE BELIEVE that IV drug use is one of the main routes of HCV transmission. However, IV drug use is only a significant route of transmission in industrialized nations, where medical procedures are usually performed with sterilized instruments under sterile conditions. Although IV drug use is a worldwide problem, from a global perspective, the use of contaminated medical equipment is by far the most common means of transmission, and IV drug use accounts for only a small proportion of the HCV infections worldwide. Approximately 10 percent of those diagnosed with HCV have no recognized source of infection.

Why IV drug users are at high risk

As we mentioned above, IV drug use accounts for only a small proportion of HCV infections worldwide. Nonetheless, hep C can be easily transmitted by sharing "works." Intravenous drug users run a high risk of contracting many diseases—including **HIV** and hepatitis B, as well as hepatitis C. When you use IV drugs, you're injecting a substance directly into your bloodstream. In most cases, you don't know what this substance contains. Moreover, since you're puncturing your skin with needles, your blood gets all over the equipment you're using. This equipment, which users call their "works," includes water, "cookers," such as spoons or anything used to "cook" drugs, and tourniquets or "ties," as well as needles. Unless you use new works each time, this equipment contains trace amounts of your blood—which you can't see. And if you share any of your works with °anyone else, their blood can get into your bloodstream and vice versa. This is one of the easiest ways to transmit blood-borne viruses like hep C, hep B, and HIV, as well as numerous other infections.

The National Institute of Drug Abuse (NIDA) says hepatitis C infection happens soon after people start using IV drugs. Fifty to 80 percent are infected within six to 12 months. Hepatitis C is actually easier to get through sharing "works" than either hep B or HIV. Unlike HIV, the hep C virus doesn't "die" when exposed to air. Recent studies suggest that HCV can survive on surfaces at room temperature at least 16 hours, but no longer than four days.[5] This is why it's dangerous to reuse equipment such as spoons that have been sitting around for a long time. Never reuse equipment—even on yourself. The virus mutates so rapidly that you can reinfect yourself with different strains of the virus.

Brief immersion in bleach does not kill HCV. If you absolutely must reuse equipment, immerse it in full-strength bleach for 20 minutes and scrub vigorously. Most household disinfectants, including full-strength bleach, will not sterilize your equipment. **Sterilization** is the process of destroying all microbial life. Even if you immerse something in bleach for 20 minutes, it may still contain some microbes. Sterilization is usually done in a hospital through moist heat by steam autoclaving, ethylene oxide gas, and dry heat.

Less common means of transmission

Hep C is most often transmitted when contaminated blood directly enters a person's arteries or veins. Nonetheless, it's important to avoid all exposure to other people's blood. Below is a list of other possible routes of transmission:

○ Sharing other kinds of drug paraphernalia, including sharing straws used for snorting speed or cocaine and sharing crack or speed pipes. These pipes get very hot, so people get burns on their lips and fingers and transmit the virus that way.
○ Sharing household items, including razors, toothbrushes, nail clippers, manicure scissors, or anything that may draw blood.
○ Needlesticks. Health care workers are especially at risk for needlestick injuries.

Sexual transmission is considered low risk. We'll discuss this further in our chapter on sex in Month 5.

A common misconception is that hep C can be caused by drinking too much alcohol. Large quantities of alcohol can cause nonviral hepatitis, but it cannot cause hepatitis C.

> *"People act so strange about hep C. It seems like they either get hysterical and think they're going to get it from the air you breathe, or they don't have a clue about basic hygiene, and they kiss a cut on your finger 'to make it better.' It's like they aren't realistic. They have no idea what a blood-borne virus is, or how you get it."*
>
> —NORA B.

> *"I spent the night at a friend's house. I had my period, and I accidentally left some bloodstains on the sheets. I had talked to my friend about hep C and the way it was transmitted. My friend called me that night. She was very upset, because she had tried to get the blood out of her sheets, but while she was scrubbing them, she realized she had tiny cuts on her hands. She called a lot of hep C hotlines. They told her that there was almost no risk involved. I was sad that she was so upset and that she was having such a strong reaction—based on so little knowledge."*
>
> —MICHELE N.

> *"A man cut his foot in the steam room of my gym. The blood was pouring out, and people were just sitting in the steam room watching it pool on the floor. I kept telling him he needed to bandage that up. Finally he walked out to the shower, tracking blood all over the floor. I went out to the front desk to get bandages for him. I told them, 'You have to mop that locker room floor with bleach. It's a health hazard.' They didn't seem to realize the urgency of it. But people walk around the locker room with athlete's foot and sores on their*

feet. I don't know how much of a risk that is, but I've heard the hep C virus can live for three to four weeks in dry blood."

—TRAVIS J.

How to prevent transmission

Once you know how hep C is transmitted, it's not hard to prevent. In the first place, make sure your family and friends know not share razors, manicure scissors, nail clippers, toothbrushes, or anything that could be contaminated with blood, even if the blood is not visible. Don't leave these items lying about where people can easily use them, especially if you have children. We discuss how to teach children to prevent the spread of hep C and other infectious disease in Month 10. Those of you who have kids or work with kids might want to read this section sooner.

Use standard precautions

You can tell your family and friends not to use your toothbrush in particular, but what if you don't feel comfortable telling them that you have hep C? You can still teach them about "standard precautions."

Standard precautions are the CDC's guidelines for preventing the transmission of blood-borne pathogens (like hep C, HIV, and hep B) in hospitals, schools, day care centers, workplaces and homes. The basic principle is to assume that everyone's blood and body fluids contain pathogens. This isn't just make-believe, because 40 to 90 percent of people with infectious diseases don't know they have them. Also, as you may know from experience, many diseases, such as viral hepatitis and HIV, are stigmatized. Those of us who have them often face discrimination and ostracism. These reactions are based on ignorance of the way infectious diseases are spread. We can't prevent diseases by excluding people, because we never know for sure who is infected and who isn't. The only way to prevent transmission is by avoiding contact with people's body fluids.

The CDC recommends wearing latex or polyurethane gloves when you come into contact with blood, feces, nasal secretions, saliva, tears, urine, or vomit—any body fluid except sweat—unless you can easily contain the fluid with a thick cloth or nonporous material. (In an emergency you can take off your coat or shirt and use that. Witnesses will think you're heroic.) You should also wear gloves when you touch people's mucous membranes, wounds, sores, or badly chapped skin, even if you don't see any blood. It's a good idea to keep a box of plastic gloves at home and in your car. You can buy latex gloves at any drugstore or medical supply store. People who are allergic to latex can use polyurethane gloves. If you don't have gloves, you can use a garbage bag or plastic sandwich bag. And whether or not you've used gloves, don't forget wash your hands after cleaning up body fluids.

We don't want to scare you. A single tear probably won't kill you. The importance of these rules is most obvious in places such as hospitals and daycare centers where nurses have to be careful not to spread diseases between patients, and spills of blood, vomit, and other body fluids are less likely to make it into paper towels or the toilet. But we all have to clean up other people's body fluids from time to time, and it's crucial to know how to do this without catching a disease. If you're not used to these precautions, they may feel awkward at first. But if you use them consistently, they will become second nature.

One advantage of standard precautions is that, if we all practice them, no one has to be singled out or treated differently because he or she has an infectious disease.

Some rules of thumb:

O Don't share razors, manicure scissors, nail clippers, toothbrushes, hairbrushes, or any other items that can break skin.

O If you use drugs, do not share any part of your works or other drug paraphernalia with other people. Inform people of the risks, or hide your equipment, if you think someone might use them.

O If you take injectable medications such as interferon or insulin, dispose of needles in sharps containers. If you don't have a sharps containers don't dump needles directly in the garbage. Put them in a soda can, and cover the opening with tape, or stuff something inside so the needle can't slip out and prick someone.

O Clean counters and floors on which body fluids have been spilled with a one-part bleach to ten-part water solution or other disinfectant.

O Discard paper towels and other materials you use to clean up the spill in a securely sealed plastic bag.

○ Avoid inoculations and surgery if you're in a part of the world where medical procedures are less likely to be performed under sterile conditions.

○ When you have to clean up a spill: if it's wet and human, don't touch it without gloves.

○ If it's wet and human and may splash or spray, protect your mucous membranes (the moist areas) of your eyes, nose, and mouth. Wear glasses, sunglasses or a facemask if possible.[6]

*"I became really sick and my doctor thought I had mono.
I couldn't get out of bed and I couldn't eat. I had never done
IV drugs or gotten a blood transfusion so my doctor thought
there was no reason to test me for hep C. But after the mono
test came back negative, he had to give it a shot. I came back
HCV positive. We went over my entire life, trying to see how
I had gotten it. I used to do a lot of cocaine, and my doctor
decided that must have been how I got it. I had no clue that
hep C could be passed by sharing straws to snort coke.
Just thinking of all of the people I have done coke with scares
me. I could have given it to hundreds of people. This disease
is really scary. It truly is an epidemic."*

—TED U.

Preventing transmission among kids

○ Get your kids tested for hep C.

○ Tell your children how hep C is transmitted, if they are old enough to understand. See Month 10 for tips on how to talk to children about hep C.

○ Put away household items that may be contaminated with your blood. This is especially important if your children are too young to understand how hep C is transmitted.

○ Some kids like to poke themselves and play with sharp objects like needles in a sewing kit. It's also popular for adolescents to pierce their ears. Explain to your kids why this is dangerous and discourage them from doing this at home with their friends. You may want to take them to a professional to get their ears pierced.

Can I get it from tattoos and piercings?

The CDC states that it is not known if there is an association between tattooing and Hep C. Any percutaneous (under the skin) exposure has the potential for transmitting blood-borne pathogens, yet there is no data that tattooing increases the risk for HCV. In the past 20 years, less than 1 percent of newly acquired HCV infections had a history of being tattooed. The CDC is currently conducting a large study to evaluate tattooing and tattoo settings as a potential risk. The only known danger is when the tattoo artist uses nonsterile equipment. It's possible to get hep C if the tattoo artist is using used needles or even used ink. If a jar of ink has had a used needle dipped in it, it's contaminated with someone's blood. As we've mentioned, the HCV virus can remain viable outside the body and can be transmitted through tiny amounts of blood.

In the United States, tattooing poses minimal risk, because tattoo parlors are required by law to use sterile needles and new jars of ink for each client. In this country, people need to be warned not to share "works" a lot more than they need to be scared of getting tattoos. Nonetheless, if you're getting a tattoo, it never hurts to ask if the parlor is using new needles and new ink for each client.

Getting your ears or any part of your body pierced in a professional setting in the United States is most likely safe. Like tattoo parlors, piercing studios have to abide by certain standards. If you are concerned, you can ask to see them use a new needle or piercing gun.

Many people, especially adolescents, pierce themselves at home or with friends and exchange earrings. We both pierced our ears countless times when we were kids. When we were growing up in the 80s it was very popular to have multiple piercings and to do them yourself. Lisa remembers being at a party with a friend who was piercing ears. Her friend was soaking the needles in some kind of household disinfectant, then using the same needles on different people. Now we know that hep C can be transmitted this way: It's crucial to use new needles on each person. As we said above, most household disinfectants do not sterilize. Rubbing alcohol is not a strong disinfectant. Its primary use is to remove oil from the skin, and even soaking a needle or earring in bleach does not guarantee that you have killed everything on it. So unless you have an autoclave in your house, don't try sterilizing at home. As we discuss earlier in this section, disinfection is not sterilization. If you have children, it's a good idea to tell them why they shouldn't pierce themselves or their friends.

Exercise

Is there any way that you might be transmitting the virus to others? What measures can you take now to prevent this from happening?

Do you need to stop sharing a razor, or hide a razor or scissors from your roommate or children? Look around your house and hide or put away anything that could be dangerous.

If you use IV drugs, can you go to a needle exchange? Can you make sure you have all the equipment you need and plenty of it, so you don't have to share or reuse?

IN A SENTENCE:

> *Hep C is transmitted blood to blood; in industrialized nations, the most common risk factors are sharing "works" and having received blood products before 1992.*

living

Telling People about Your Hep C

"When I found out that I had hep C, I was so upset. I rushed home and immediately told my partner. It was like a contact fear. She became just as distraught as I was. Neither of us knew anything about the disease. I wish the doctor had given me more information that I could have given to her."

—FRANK MILES

"I am very out about my hep C. It hasn't always been this way. I know I got hep C from using IV drugs, and at first I was ashamed. Then I figured, who cares? It was something I did, and now I'm paying for it. So many of us have hep C. If we all come out of the closet, then maybe something will be done about it. We can't simply sit in silence forever."

—KIM L.

COMMUNICATION IS essential to any relationship, whether you're ordering dinner or talking to your partner of fifty years. Throughout this book we discuss communication in relation to various topics, including long-term partnerships, your social life, dating, and raising children. This chapter will help you decide who needs to know about your diagnosis right away, what to tell them, and how.

Whom to tell right away

"When I first got my hep C diagnosis, I sat down and thought about whom I wanted to tell. After making a few lists I decided that I didn't want to live that way. I wanted to tell everyone. After all, I have always been a very open person. I am not ashamed of having hep C. There is nothing wrong with me. I just happen to provide a home for a virus. I hear about people talking about me behind my back. Sometimes my friends ask me why I tell people if it's just going to make my life harder. But you know what? In the long run, the more people who know about hep C, the more people will demand something be done about it. And that is one of the only things that can make my life easier."

—Tom L.

When you find out you have hep C, your first impulse may be to talk about the diagnosis with anyone who will listen, but it is important to exercise great care in deciding whom to tell. Once you share information with someone, you can never take it back. Telling one person is often tantamount to telling everyone. It's a good idea to tell all your health care providers. This is generally safe because they have an ethical obligation to protect their patients' privacy. Whom you tell is your decision. But there are some people you might want to tell immediately.

Deciding whom to tell and what to tell them

It's likely that the first people you tell will be some of the most important people in your life. What you say depends on the person and your relationship to them. Ask yourself whom you need to tell for your own emotional well-being. Is it your best friend? Your mother? Your therapist?

Whom do you need to talk to? This is a balancing act too. If you're feeling emotionally fragile, you may need to ask yourself who will be able to listen sympathetically and who will be supportive. Has this person responded compassionately to people with HIV or other illnesses?

Telling long-term partners and spouses

If you have a long-term partner or spouse, you will most likely want to tell that person. Remember, the virus can't be transmitted through hugging or kissing, unless both people have bleeding gums or an open mouth sore, which could allow blood-to-blood contact. Studies have failed to detect the presence of HCV in saliva, semen, or urine. According to the CDC and Melissa Palmer, M.D., sex is an extremely inefficient means of transmission. Experts at the Mayo Clinic say that if you're in a long-term monogamous relationship with someone who has hep C, your risk is 0 to 0.6 percent per year. If you're in a short-term relationship and your partner has hep C, your risk is 1 percent per year, and the CDC recommends routine condom use. This risk increases if your partner is HIV-positive.[3]

Despite the low rate of sexual transmission, your long-term partner is likely to have emotional reactions. Your partner might fear having contracted it from you, and might be angry if that is the case. Whether or not your partner is concerned about his or her own hep C status, he or she will most likely be upset to learn that you have a chronic illness. It's a good idea to break it to him or her gently in order to give time to process the information.

Despite the low risk of sexual transmission, it's also a good idea for your long-term partners to be tested. If your partner tests positive, don't assume that he or she got it from you, or vice versa. Many HCV-positive partners even have different genotypes of the virus, which shows that they have different sources of infection.

Even if you're sure that one of you infected the other, it's important not to cast blame, or take on responsibility for something you have no control over. Remember that in the scheme of things hep C is a recently discovered illness, and you can't hold people responsible for not telling you about something they didn't know about.

Telling parents and caretakers

"When my daughter first called and told me she had hepatitis C, I was devastated. We ordered a book and read the entire thing in one night. The stories were so depressing. I cried for days. I was so worried that she was never going to have a normal life. She is only 27. I want her to be able to accomplish everything she has dreamed about. The entire family became proactive in learning about the disease, and now we are all dealing with her hep C better."

—MOM

"One of my daughters has had Graves Disease for about three years, then this year we found out my other daughter has hep C. It's hard as a parent to know that both your children are sick. They both handle it well. But as a parent, it's impossible for me not to worry."

—DIANE B.

Be gentle with your parents. It may be really hard for them to know that you're suffering or to think that they may have to watch you die before them. This is a lifelong illness, and it will bring up life and death issues. They may go into complete denial, or they may want to take care of you in a way that seems suffocating. Their reactions may not be what you expect or want, but remember that, however they react, it's probably hard for them. They're going through a grief process just as you are. Give them time. Unless you're really sick, you and your parents will have time to process your feelings, and you don't have to resolve everything right away.

Talking to your children

If you want to talk to your children now, you can skip ahead to the chapter on children in Month 10. The important thing to do right away is to hide your razors, manicure scissors, and anything else they might get into that could have your blood on it. Depending on the age of your child, protect-ing them may be more important than telling them. It's up to you to decide at what age they're mature enough to understand. As we emphasize in Month 3, it's best to exercise caution in telling schools, day care centers, and other parents about a child's hep C. You don't want your child singled out or ostracized. As long as schools and day care centers are using stan-dard precautions, you may not need to tell them.

Telling your friends

It's important to be able to ask your friends for emotional and other types of support. You might need people to talk to, and you might also need practical help getting to the doctor or other appointments. However, when you've just found out you have hep C, you may not want to tell everyone right away. You may want to consider whom you trust and who will be supportive. Some of your friends may not react the way you would like them to. It is hard for most people to hear that someone close to them is sick. Be sure to give people time and help them to understand that they are not at risk and that you are not going to die tomorrow.

If you use or have used IV drugs

If you know people who have used IV drugs, we encourage you to tell them that they're at high risk for hep C and let them know how it is trans-mitted. This can be especially difficult if you have done IV drugs yourself and have shared works with these people. In this case, it's possible that you contracted the virus from them, or they contracted it from you. If you still use, the most important thing you can do is make sure that no one ever uses your equipment and that you never use theirs.

IN A SENTENCE:

It's your decision whom you tell about your hep C.

learning

Communication Tips for Talking about Your Diagnosis

HERE ARE some communication tips for telling people about your diagnosis. We use these techniques ourselves, and they may help you when you first begin coming out to people about your hep C. Since this is a lifelong illness, you'll most likely be doing this for, well, the rest of your life. It will get easier as you go along, and we'll be coming back to the topic of communication throughout this book.

- ○ Know what you want from the conversation.
- ○ Ask yourself what you hope to accomplish.
- ○ Identify your needs and ask for what you need. Do you want a load off your mind? Do you want sympathy? Support? What kind of support?
- ○ Be clear why you think this information is important to the person you're telling. Ask yourself why the person needs to know. Is he or she at risk?

○ Plan ahead for the right place at the right time.
○ Find a time that's good for both of you. You might want to tell them in advance that you have something important to tell them and ask when they would be available to hear it.
○ Find a private place where you can have a comfortable conversation.
○ Be informed.
○ Bring books or pamphlets on hep C. The person you tell may have some urgent questions like: Are you going to die? Am I at risk? What's going to happen to you? Are you going to get very sick? Whether you're concerned about putting the person at ease or convincing him or her to get tested, the more informed you are and the more information you bring with you the better. It's a good idea to bring a book like this one that has an index, so that you can look up information if you need to. Even if you're well informed, it will validate what you're saying.

What to tell people

○ Risk factors: Tell people how the virus is transmitted and how it's not transmitted.
○ Be sure to tell your friends and loved ones that they can't get it through kissing, hugging, sharing glasses, or casual contact. You may also want to share the statistics on sexual transmission with current or potential partners.
○ If you know the person you're telling has used IV drugs, it's important to be very specific about the risk factors in sharing works. You can get across how important it is to be tested by telling him or her that the vast majority of IV drug users have this virus.

You can't control someone else's reactions

Even though you can't foresee how people will respond to what you tell them, it helps not to be thrown off guard. Be prepared for some of the following possible reactions.

"How did you get that?"

When someone asks you how you got hep C, keep in mind that most people ask this question innocently. They most likely want to know how the virus is transmitted, so they can avoid getting it themselves.

Nonetheless, many people with hep C feel as if this question is nosy and impolite. Most of us don't know exactly how we got the disease, and even if we do, we might not want to tell people we don't know well. Some of us feel as if the person asking the question is blaming us for the fact that we have this disease—especially since many people associate hep C with IV drug use. We may think they're asking if we've used IV drugs, or assuming that we must have done something bad if we have hep C. This stigma can be painful, even if you know you got hep C from a blood transfusion. If you did in fact get hep C from sharing "works," you may feel uncomfortable answering this question truthfully. That's a perfectly valid feeling. You don't have to tell anyone you don't want to. As we've said before, no matter how you got hep C, you don't deserve this illness. You come first. Take care of yourself, deal with your own feelings, and talk to people who are going to be supportive, before you tell people who are going to guilt trip you.

"Did I get it from you?"

You may think that another person contracted hep C from you. It's possible that he or she did, if you donated blood for this person before 1992, if the two of you have shared IV needles or other works, or even if you've shared household items that may have been contaminated with your blood.

If you need to tell someone that they may have contracted hep C from you, it's important to break it to them gently and be prepared to deal with their anger. In this situation, you may also be experiencing a lot of guilt, especially if the two of you have done IV drugs together. If you had no idea you had hep C, you're not responsible for the fact that someone else may have gotten it from you. Unless you stuck a needle in someone else's arm, they made a decision to do IV drugs and to share works with you, and this decision entails a risk of exposure to blood-borne pathogens. Both of you were taking a big risk, because either of you could have contracted a disease from the other. While you may still feel guilty, it's important to remember that everyone is responsible for making his or her own decisions, and we all make choices we regret later. You are not responsible for someone else's choices and actions.

"Can I get it from you?"

The answer to this question is "It's extremely unlikely, unless we have blood-to-blood contact." You may need to inform this person that HCV can survive household disinfectants and tell him or her about less common means of blood-to-blood transmission, such as razors and manicure scissors. If you know how hep C is transmitted, it's relatively easy to prevent transmission. Don't be alarmed if friends who you've only hugged, kissed, or shared a glass with you ask if they can get hep C from you. It's most likely not because they think you're dirty, but just because they're not informed. They might be confusing hep C with hep A, which you can get from food and casual contact. Once again, the best way to respond to this question is to be informed.

Sexual partners are also likely to ask about transmission risks. When you tell them, it's a good idea to have some information with you. In this case, statistics can be very reassuring. See Month 5, "Yes, You Can Have Sex," for more information. You can also refer them to the CDC's "Frequently Asked Questions about Hepatitis C" at http://0-www.cdc.gov.mill1.sj library.org/ncidod/diseases/hepatitis/c/faq.htm#1b1. If your partner can't get past the fear or even listen to the information, then maybe you should find someone else. Chances are you will have chronic hep C, and you need someone who will be there to support you. It's hard enough having a chronic illness alone, but it may be even harder having one when you're in a relationship with someone who isn't there for you.

"I told my partner that I'd tested positive for HCV, and that I thought I'd gotten it from him. He said he didn't have it. I said how do you know? And he said, I just know."

—LAUREN L.

"When I told my parents that I had hep C they asked me how I think I could have gotten it. I told them honestly—that I

*used to use drugs. They were devastated. They told me that
getting this disease is my fault, and that there was nothing
they could do to help me. I need their help now more than I
ever have. I wish I hadn't told them the truth."*

—EDWARD D.

Special circumstances

In Day 1 we encouraged you to focus on the present and not on how you
got hep C. Unless you know that you received contaminated blood products, it may be hard to pinpoint the exact date or circumstances surrounding your infection. The more important question is how you can live
a healthy life, now that you have it.

On the other hand, you may have a very good idea about how you contracted hep C and whom you got it from. If you want to talk to this person
about it, it's important to know what you need out of the conversation. Be
sure you're not scapegoating someone. Be clear about what's your responsibility and what's theirs. Unless someone deliberately stuck a needle in
your arm, it's unlikely that one person is entirely responsible for "giving you"
hep C. Nonetheless, you may feel as if the person omitted information
about his or her hep C status. You may want an apology, or you may want
reassurance that the person did not know he or she had hep C and did not
give it to you knowingly. You may need to get things out in the open and talk
about how you feel.

If you want to talk to someone who may have infected you, here are
some suggestions for how to get information across in a way that he or she
can hear it.

Use "I" instead of "you." Unless you want to get into a fight, you'll get
a lot further in your conversation if you avoid accusations and demands such
as "You gave me the virus!" or "You should get tested!" The words "you" and
"should" are red flags. If you say "You gave this to me!" you're likely to get a
response of denial or anger: "I did not." If you want to get the information
across, it is best to speak in "I" statements like "I'm concerned you may be
at risk" or "I just found out I tested positive for hep C. I'm concerned about
what we've done together. Have you been tested?" Remember, you can't

make someone get tested. That's a person's own responsibility. The most you can do is tell the person in a way he or she can hear.

Try not to tell people what to do. Think in terms of making suggestions, rather than giving advice. When you're talking about your feelings, it's especially important to use "I" statements. Instead of saying "you're making me feel guilty," say "I feel guilty." You can't make somebody feel a certain way. No one has that kind of control over other people's feelings and reactions.

There's a good chance that the person who "gave" you hep C didn't know she had it and may not know anything about the disease. In that case it's important to tell him or her how it's transmitted so he or she can take care in the future to avoid giving it to someone else. You may feel the need to let him or her know how upset you are and the importance of getting tested. The situation is much more complicated if the person who gave you hep C knew he or she may have had the virus and was in denial about it, or didn't take the proper precautions to prevent transmitting it to you. In this circumstance, you may have different needs and feelings. You may, for instance, want him or her to acknowledge the severity of what he's done and be much more careful in the future.

"When I received my hepatitis C diagnosis, my doctor asked me if I had ever shot IV drugs. I had been using drugs with my boyfriend and my doctor told me that was most likely how I got it. I had asked my boyfriend when we started using drugs if he had been tested and what the results were. He had assured me that he had been tested and was fine. When I told him about my diagnosis that evening, he didn't seem surprised. When I talked to one of his former girlfriends, she told me that he had received a positive hep C diagnosis years earlier. I was devastated. I confronted him about this, and he denied her accusations, telling me that he had received one positive diagnosis and then two negative ones. He blew off my diagnosis, telling me it was 'no big deal' and 'not the end of the world.' I needed him to tell me that he knew he gave me the virus. I needed to hear it for two

reasons: one, for my own peace of mind, and two, to have him realize the severity of what he had done in the hope that he would never do it to someone else."

—AMY C.

In such a case you may feel a need to warn other people who might be in danger. This is a hard call. Remember that this is others' responsibility and not yours.

Exercise

- ○ Make a list of the people you need to tell, if anyone.
- ○ Collect information on hep C to give people.
- ○ Call one of the people on your list and make a time that's convenient for both of you to talk.

IN A SENTENCE:

When telling people about your hep C, it's good to know what you want from the conversation and be informed.

living

Symptoms You Might Be Experiencing

"When I tell people I have fatigue, they don't understand what I'm talking about. They think that I am just tired. Like sleep or coffee will fix me. Fatigue is a lot different from being tired. Fatigue is something that you feel in your entire body. It's hard to do anything. You are exhausted to the core. You can't just go to sleep and wake up cured. There is nothing that helps but time."

—LIZA B.

"My boyfriend was so healthy when I met him. He was an athlete, and he was in really good shape. Within a year he was sick with hep C. He'd most likely had it for over 20 years. He'd gotten non-A-non-B hepatitis in the 70s. He had gotten really sick and almost died, but then he had gotten

*better, and he didn't realize that he had a chronic condition.
The first sign that something was wrong was that his legs
would swell up. By the time we found out that he had hep C
his liver was cirrhotic."*

—JOHN H.

PEOPLE WITH hep C report a wide range of symptoms—ranging from mild fatigue to debilitating illness. Many people are **asymptomatic**, and some of the most common symptoms, such as mild fatigue and depression, occur so frequently in people without hep C that it's hard to say whether or not the virus is causing them. Most people don't experience any severe symptoms for 20 to 30 years, and as many as 80 percent will most likely outlive the disease and die from an unrelated cause. The slow progress of the disease and lack of symptoms are two reasons why hep C is called the "silent epidemic." Many people live for years—even their entire lives—without knowing they have hep C. They never get tested, because they don't think there's anything wrong with them. This can be misleading and deadly. Some people with severe liver damage experience no symptoms. Fortunately, your doctor can monitor the health of your liver with some of the tests described in the Learning section of this chapter. Your symptoms or lack thereof are not a direct indicator of the severity of disease or degree of damage.

Most commonly reported symptoms

Many people with hep C report some or all of the following symptoms.

- ○ Fatigue
- ○ Depression
- ○ Joint pains
- ○ Flulike symptoms, including nausea, chills, and fever
- ○ "Brain fog"
- ○ Decreased libido
- ○ Swelling and pain in the region of the liver
- ○ Irritable bowel syndrome
- ○ Bloating
- ○ Menstrual difficulties, severe PMS

- ○ Sleep disorders
- ○ Bruising and bleeding easily
- ○ Itchy skin
- ○ Adverse reaction to drinking alcohol

With or without hep C, you've most likely experienced most of these symptoms at some point in your life. They are not always related to hep C, and they don't necessarily indicate liver damage. Many of these complaints can be alleviated by stress reduction, rest, and changes in diet, exercise, and lifestyle. Unfortunately some people with hep C experience extreme versions of these symptoms, such as debilitating fatigue. It's important not to deny your own symptoms or anyone else's. Just because you have never had a problem doesn't mean that other people's symptoms aren't valid.

The symptoms listed above are not the most widely known symptoms of hepatitis. When most people think of hepatitis, they think of **jaundice**, the buildup of **bilirubin** that makes you skin turn yellow. Bilirubin is the yellowish pigment produced in the breakdown of red blood cells. This breakdown first produces hemoglobin, and its major component is converted into bilirubin. The liver recycles bilirubin into **bile**. A high level of bilirubin may indicate that too many red blood cells are dying. The buildup of bilirubin in the skin causes jaundice, a common symptom of hepatitis A and B.

Only 20 to 30 percent of people with HCV experience jaundice. Some people may not believe you have hepatitis because you aren't yellow. Sharing information about HCV may help them understand what you're going through.

> *"I always thought that having hepatitis meant that you were going to turn yellow. I wasn't yellow. I wasn't anything. But suddenly I was just another person with hep C."*
>
> —NINA G.

> *"I was talking to a friend of mine who has lupus. There are many similarities between our diseases—we are both fatigued, have joint pain, and have trouble sleeping. Yet when I told her that I thought they were similar, she snapped at me. She said that her disease drastically affected her life*

and mine didn't. She said that I had an 'easy' disease, and that I should quit complaining."

—CARLA T.

"I am sure I feel pain in my liver. My doctor told me that's impossible because the liver doesn't feel pain. Now I feel crazy. Am I causing myself some psychosomatic pain? Am I driving myself crazy?"

—LOUIS D.

Exercise

Use your journal to record any symptoms you're experiencing, even if they may not be related to hep C.

Classic symptoms of acute hepatitis

○ A protracted and severe flulike illness. This often includes extreme fatigue, anorexia (decreased hunger), nausea, abdominal pain, joint pain, fevers and chills.

○ Dark urine. The liver is not properly filtering toxins, so the urine contains extra bilirubin, a breakdown product of hemoglobin, which would normally go into the stool.

○ Light stool. There are fewer byproducts of hemoglobin breakdown in the stool and there is fat in the stool as well. A healthy liver excretes bile into the intestines. This bile breaks down fats so that you can absorb them. In acute hepatitis, the liver may be unable to make bile acids necessary to absorb fat, so fat comes out in the stool.

○ **Jaundice**. The buildup of bilirubin in the skin turns the eyes and skin yellow.

Although these symptoms are most often associated with HAV and HBV, 10 to 20 percent of those infected with HCV experience a bout of acute hepatitis several months following exposure. This is called a seroconversion illness.

Seroconversion illness

Some people experience a protracted flulike illness approximately six weeks to three months following exposure to HCV. Seroconversion is the body's process of mounting an immune response and producing antibodies to hepatitis C. At the end of this process, the patient tests positive for HCV antibodies.

- ○ The average seroconversion time is eight to nine weeks.
- ○ 80 percent have detectable antibodies within 15 weeks following exposure.
- ○ Over 90 percent seroconvert within five months, and
- ○ 97 percent by six months.

Some people have symptoms before they test positive for antibodies. If you have symptoms and are at risk for HCV, you might want to ask your doctor to test you for HCV RNA, which will be present in the blood before antibodies.

Many people never experience a seroconversion illness, or don't realize that they're having a bout of hepatitis.

- ○ 60 to 70 percent have no symptoms.
- ○ 20 to 30 percent have jaundice.
- ○ 10 to 20 percent experience nonspecific symptoms such as malaise, anorexia, nausea, and vomiting.

Lisa and Cara both experienced acute seroconversion illnesses. Lisa thought she had the worst flu she'd ever had. Cara was throwing up constantly and so weak she couldn't get out of bed. In some cases the symptoms are milder, and some recreational and pharmaceutical drugs can mask this illness as well.

"I have been going through a seroconversion illness almost all year. My doctor tells me that this is a good thing. That my body is initiating an immune response to the hepatitis. I know a few other people who have had seroconversion illnesses as well, but most people don't and many people don't

believe me. I am coming out of it now and have more good days than bad. But I am not 100 percent better. Some days I am extremely fatigued, as in whole body fatigue, and often my legs hurt. I seem to hold all my pain in my legs."

—TINA S.

Most people who suffer seroconversion symptoms recover within a few months. After the acute infection, 15 to 25 percent are thought to resolve the infection, meaning that no HCV is detected in the blood, and liver tests return to normal. In most cases, however, laboratory tests show persistent or fluctuating liver tests, indicating viral activity. We describe these tests in the following section.

IN A SENTENCE:

> *Many people with hep C are asymptomatic for 20 to 30 years.*

learning

Your Test Results and What They Mean

"My tests are so confusing. I've always been scared of numbers, and I don't know what they mean. The scariest part is how wildly they fluctuate. I feel like my doctor never has time to go over each test with me."

—BILL J.

WHEN YOU were diagnosed with hep C, your doctor probably gave you a variety of blood tests. If he gave you a copy of your test results, go get them now, so you can follow along as we explain those letters and numbers. If not, be sure to call your doctor and request copies of all your blood work. You will be getting some of these tests at least every six months for many years to come. It's a good idea to set up a file now and keep track of all your test results. Lisa has her results dating back to 1990. You need a doctor to interpret your blood work, but don't rely on your doctor to keep track of all your results. Keep copies of your own medical records. When you go to another doctor or a liver specialist, you may have to take copies of your test results with you.

Get your liver panels every three months

One of the most important things you can do for yourself is to get regular blood tests called liver panels. Your doctor can use these tests to assess the damage that hepatitis C might be doing to your liver and how well the liver is performing its functions. It's a good idea to get these tests every three months for the first two years after you're diagnosed. After that you can get them every six months.

Liver enzyme tests

Two of the most common tests that doctors use to monitor their hep C patients are **ALT** and **AST**, which stand for alanine aminotransferase (ALT) and aspartate aminotransferase (AST). These sound like scary monsters, but they are enzymes in your liver cells. When liver cells die, they release ALT and AST into the bloodstream. When a person's liver cells are not being killed off by a virus or toxic substance, ALT and AST levels are usually under 30 for men and under 27 for women. According to some laboratories, the "normal range" for ALT and AST may be as high as 60. However, the word "normal" means the result of a statistical average. "Normal" ALT/AST levels are determined by taking an average from a sampling of people, some of whom have high enzymes from drinking, being infected with hep C, or some other cause. Healthy ALT and AST levels are under 30.

Most people with hep C have slightly elevated liver enzymes. This means that your liver cells are dying at a rate that is slightly higher than average. In general, the higher your enzymes are, the more active the virus is, and the more liver cells it's killing.

Nonetheless, elevated ALT and AST do not necessarily indicate the presence of the HCV virus. The enzyme levels in your blood fluctuate throughout the day, and they can be high if you had alcohol the night before or consumed some other liver-toxic substance. Any inflammation of liver cells can raise enzyme levels. See Day 7 Learning for a list of medications that can be toxic to your liver.

ALT and AST are not a reliable measure of how much damage has been done to the liver, unless they are as high as 20,000, which can happen in acute cases of Tylenol poisoning. People with cirrhosis can have normal liver enzymes, and about 30 percent of people with HCV have normal enzymes. Most people with hep C have slightly elevated enzymes, which fluctuate during the course of the day. Many doctors advise their patients not to worry unless their enzymes increase by fivefold: from 60 to 300, for instance. You need a doctor to interpret your test results in conjunction with other tests, such as a liver biopsy.

The liver also produces the enzymes **ALK** and **GGT**. **Alkaline phosphatase (ALK)** is a liver enzyme that activates the metabolism of phosphorus and delivers energy to cells in the body. Abnormal ALK may indicate bile duct blockage or alcohol or drug induced hepatitis. **Gamma-Glutamyl transpeptidase (GGT)** is an enzyme that helps in the metabolism of glutamate. Your liver panel should include tests that measure the level of these enzymes. ALK and GGT are usually not elevated unless a person has developed cirrhosis or a problem with the **biliary tract**—the ducts that drain bile from the liver into the intestine.

> *"My liver enzymes are all over the map. They seem to fluctuate with each test, and my mood goes up and down with them. My doctor told me not to worry unless the difference is more than five times."*
>
> —ROSE D.

The most important tests for monitoring the progression of liver disease

While the ALT and AST can indicate cell damage, several other tests are more reliable for monitoring the progression of liver disease. Doctors use the following tests to monitor liver functions and the progression of liver disease:

○ **Bilirubin**: The level of bilirubin indicates the overall function of the liver and health of the bile duct.

○ **Albumin**: a blood protein produced by the liver. Albumin maintains the volume of blood in blood vessels by absorbing fluid (salt and water). Low albumin level may cause fluid to leak out of arteries and veins into tissues and cause swelling, called **edema**.

○ **Prothrombin time (PT)**: Prothrombin is a protein that helps the blood clot. The test for **prothrombin time** measures how long the blood takes to clot. When the liver is not functioning well, blood clotting as measured by PT may be slower, and the person will bleed and bruise easily.

Albumin and prothrombin time are the most important tests for monitoring the progression of liver disease.

Tests for antibodies: Have you been exposed to HCV?

Before your doctor diagnosed you with hep C, she gave you an "**anti-HCV antibody test**"—that is, a test to see if you had **antibodies** to the HCV virus. A "positive" or "reactive" test indicates that you have been exposed to HCV, and your body has mounted a defense by producing antibodies. The antibody test indicates past or present infection. It does not indicate whether the virus is present in your body. Even if your body has successfully eliminated HCV, you will probably still test positive for antibodies. This makes it hard to know whether you have actually "cleared" the virus. Many doctors will tell you that you have "cleared" the virus if you have no viral load. However, viral load may come back. Many people have had no viral load for years, but at this point, not enough is known about the virus to be able to tell if these people are actually "cured." Until we know more, it's safest to live as if you have it and take precautions not to pass it to anyone else.

The most widely used antibody test is called the **anti-HCV ELISA 3** or **EIA**. **ELISA** stands for "enzyme-linked immunosorbent assay," and **EIA** for "enzyme immunoassay." The ELISA 3 is not foolproof, so the results need to be confirmed by another test.

Tests that tell whether the virus is detectable in your blood

If you test positive for HCV antibodies, your doctor may give you a PCR test (polymerase chain reaction) to confirm that the virus is present in your bloodstream.

Many laboratories now use the HCV RNA PCR test after the ELISA 3 then follow up with the RIBA 3 (Recombinant Immunoblot Assay) if the HCV RNA test is negative and the ELISA 3 test is positive. Blood banks also use the RIBA 3 to confirm a positive ELISA 3. The best approach to confirm the diagnosis of hepatitis C is to test for HCV RNA using a sensitive assay such as polymerase chain reaction (PCR) or transcription-mediated amplification (TMA). The presence of HCV RNA in serum indicates an active infection. HCV RNA testing is also necessary for immunocompromised patients who may have trouble producing HCV antibodies or people who are experiencing an acute HCV infection.

Testing has advanced so much in recent years that people at risk for hep C who tested negative in the past should get tested again.

There are two types of PCR tests. The qualitative test simply indicates whether HCV genetic material (HCV RNA) is detectable in your blood. The quantitative PCR test measures the amount of HCV RNA in your blood and translates it into the number of units of virus per milliliter of blood. This number is your viral load. Viral loads for people with hep C can range from "undetectable" to 100 million IU/milliliter. There is now a standard unit of measurement for HCV RNA: the International Unit (IU).

The quantitative PCR test is somewhat limited as a diagnostic tool, because your viral load can fluctuate dramatically, increasing by tenfold if your liver or immune system is under stress. The PCR test also has a 5 percent rate of false negatives, because the viral load may be at too low a level to measure. Researchers have recently developed more sensitive viral load tests. Currently available PCR assays will detect HCV RNA in serum down to a lower limit of 50 to 100 copies per milliliter (mL), which is equivalent to 25 to 50 international units (IU). A slightly more sensitive TMA test has recently become available. Between 50 and 2,000 is very low, 1 to 2 million is medium, 2 to 25 million is high, and over 25 million is very high. Viral load does not correlate with the severity of your condition or prognosis, but there may be a correlation between viral load and treatment with antiviral therapy.[1]

> *"I got my first viral load test. I have a lot of friends who have HIV, and I'm used to hearing their viral loads. When I heard I had a viral load of over 10 million, I thought I was a goner, because someone who had this load with HIV would be long gone by now. Then I heard that that was actually pretty standard for people with hep C. It's amazing how much less lethal this virus is than the HIV virus."*
>
> —DAVE N.

Genotypes: The genetic variations of HCV

Due to the virus's high mutation rate, there are 6 basic **genotypes**, or genetic variations, and 50 subtypes.

- O Genotype 1a is mostly found in North and South America and Australia.
- O Genotype 1b is prevalent in North America, Europe, and Japan.
- O Genotype 2a is mainly found in China and Japan.
- O Genotype 2b is the most common subtype of 2 in the United States and Northern Europe. It also occurs in Japan, Taiwan, and China.
- O Genotype 2c is the subtype of 2 most common in Western and Southern Europe.
- O Genotype 3 is common in Scotland and throughout the UK, Europe, and to a lesser extent in the United States.
- O Genotype 3a predominates in Australia and southern Asia.
- O Genotype 4 is prevalent in the Middle East and in Northern and Central Africa.
- O Genotype 4a is most common is Egypt. There is a high incidence of 4c in Central Africa
- O Genotype 5a is mostly confined to South Africa.
- O Genotype 6 occurs mainly in Asia, particularly Hong Kong. Genotype 6a is restricted to Hong Kong, Macau, and Vietnam.

Your doctor may give you a genotype test to determine whether your infection is likely to respond to interferon-based drug therapy. Types 2 and 3 are very effectively treated by interferon/ribavirin combination therapy. Unfortunately, Type 1a, which is the most common in the U.S., is also the most resistant to all currently approved forms of treatment.

"I have a binder that I put all my test results in. This way I can review them easily and see how I'm doing. It helps me feel as if I'm in control of my health, at least a little bit. And at this point, any little bit helps."

—KATIE W.

Liver biopsy:
The "gold standard" for evaluating liver damage

The liver biopsy is the most widely used tool for diagnosing and evaluating liver damage. Some doctors recommend a biopsy every three to five years if you are HCV positive. Other doctors don't recommend a biopsy unless you're considering treatment. You may want to schedule a biopsy anyway to find out the extent of damage to your liver.

A biopsy is a relatively simple surgical procedure, where the doctor inserts a needle between your ribs, extracts 1/50,000th of the liver and examines the tissue under a microscope to see if fibrosis or cirrhosis is present. The grade of inflammation and the stage of fibrosis are each measured separately on a 0 to 4 scale. Fibrosis is considered mild when it is limited to the portal and periportal regions of the liver. Scar tissue that extends from one portal region to another is called "bridging fibrosis" and is considered more advanced. Patients at stage 2 or 3 are often considered good candidates for treatment.

The biopsy generally requires a four- to six-hour hospital stay but not an overnight visit. It is relatively safe and painless, with a mortality rate of only one in 9,000. Before your biopsy, ask a friend or family member to drive you home from the hospital and stay with you overnight. Lisa has had four biopsies in the 17 years she has had hep C. They were relatively painless, and she went about her regular business the next day.

More tests: Ultrasound and CT scan

The ultrasound and CT scan are nonintrusive but less accurate than the liver biopsy. An ultrasound machine translates sound waves that bounce off your organs into visual images. In a CT scan, low-level radiation offers a more detailed image of a cross section of a person's body.

Both tests look for changes in the size and structure of the liver. While a healthy liver is smooth, a cirrhotic liver is generally collapsed and covered with nodules, making it appear bumpy. These imaging tests also detect the growth of tumors and changes in the portal vein and hepatic artery. This is especially important, since blockage of the portal vein can lead to some of the most severe symptoms of liver disease.

IN A SENTENCE:

> *For the first year, it's important to get liver panels every three months.*

DAY **5**

living

Taking Care of Yourself: Minimizing Commitments and Responsibilities

"I have always been a Type A personality. I work all of the time and usually take on more than I can handle. But I'm starting to get sick from my hepatitis. At first I was very frustrated, because I couldn't do everything I wanted to do. But I had no choice but to slow down. Once I started to slow down, I realized that I was happier that way—that I really wanted to do things other than work. My life is actually a bit better now that I'm taking it easy. I don't feel as if my hep C has saved my life, but it sure has changed it."

—PAM F.

"I live with my extended family, and we're a tightly knit bunch. When we found out I had hep C, they were all over me, wanting to take care of me and make sure I was okay. It was driving me up the

wall. I realized what I really needed was time for myself. I took off a week from work, and I found a place to house-sit so I could be alone for a while."

—HEATHER S.

YOU'VE MADE it through your first four days of knowing you have hep C, but if you're like most of us, you're still feeling the shock. Being diagnosed with hep C can cause a lot of additional stress in your life. Whether you're sick or not, you may have to take some time for yourself to deal with your diagnosis. Many of us are overcommitted in both our work and social lives. If you feel incredibly overwhelmed, you may want to take a look at your commitments and decide which mean the most to you and which you can do without. You can resume these activities later, but it's important to take time for yourself to process your diagnosis. You may have to schedule some hours to do nothing. There is nothing wrong with this. You also may have to put aside some extra time to deal with the important people in your life. Everyone who cares about you will be affected by your diagnosis, and it may be a good idea to schedule time to spend with the people you love.

In some ways, hep C can be an important lesson. We were both Type A personalities who worked a lot. We still do, but we also relax and have fun. Both of us have found that having a chronic illness makes us rethink our priorities and enjoy our lives.

In order to prioritize your commitments, you first need to figure out in which areas of your life you feel fulfilled and in which you feel lacking.

Rate from zero to ten how fulfilled you feel in the following areas of your life. Zero is completely unsatisfied. Ten is completely fulfilled.

- ○ Career
- ○ Family
- ○ Close friendships
- ○ Social life
- ○ Love life
- ○ Sex life
- ○ Spirituality
- ○ Health: diet and exercise
- ○ Recreation: adventure, non-work-related creative activity, sports.

Now list your commitments in each of these areas. Put them in order of importance. Circle the ones you can't do without: What's necessary for your livelihood or personal fulfillment? Underline the ones that you need to do but wish you didn't have to do. Cross out the ones you don't need to do.

It's important to be able to say no. You don't have to say yes to everything. None of us can do everything, and you'll feel far more frustrated if you try, especially in times of great stress and fatigue.

Reducing stress: Learning to check in with your body

"I never paid attention to my body. I'm a computer programmer, and I lived for a long time as just a brain floating in space. I'm in my late 20s and just found out I had hep C. A friend of mine recommended yoga, which I thought was 'out there.' Now I get up at six a.m. and go to a yoga class. It's changed my life."

—BOB E.

Stress can weaken your immune system. It can make you more susceptible to illness and exacerbate conditions you already have. The good news is that there's a lot you can do to reduce the stress in your life. You can get in a Jacuzzi or steam bath, get a massage, do some kind of exercise you like, or make time to lie down or take a nap during the day. But we have found that one of the least time-consuming and least costly ways to reduce stress is simply to take a few minutes to notice where you are holding tension in your body. Below is a technique that works for us; we try to do this at least once a day, when we remember. The next time you're feeling stressed out, stop and ask yourself:

○ Which parts of your body feel tense?
○ Do you feel tension in your shoulders?
○ Are you holding your breath?
○ Are your feet aching?
○ Are you clenching your jaw?
○ Are you slouched over?

In time, you will develop your own set of questions, based on your own body. Once you figure out where you're holding tension, ask yourself what you can do to relax that part of your body. Here are some ideas:

O Take a few deep breaths.
O Adjust your posture or sitting position.
O Focus on the tense part of your body and try to relax it.
O Do some stretches.
O Lie down or be alone for a few minutes.

In short, checking in with your body means taking inventory of every part, noticing how it's feeling, locating areas of tension, and figuring out how you can alleviate that tension. This is a good way to reduce your stress level before it gets unbearable. You may also find that it relieves mild fatigue and depression, simply by helping you feel more relaxed throughout the day.

Remember to breathe

Breathing and consciousness of our breath is the key to relaxation and bodily awareness. Many of us hold our breath while we're talking, eating, exercising, or experiencing anxiety or stress. If we can remember to breathe through all these situations, we can reduce our stress and increase our level of energy. There are many breathing techniques, which you can explore. Here are three basic exercises to get you started:

O Place your hands on your abdomen. Allow your abdomen to swell as you inhale. The idea here is not to tighten your stomach. We're taught to hold in our stomachs, but this can constrict breathing.
O Lie down, close your eyes, or get into a meditative position and focus on your breathing. Eventually your mind will start to wander. This is normal, but try to bring your mind back gently without beating yourself up about it. Try doing this for five minutes at first. Then gradually increase the time.
O Imagine that you are breathing into a part of your body that is tense or in pain. See if you can soothe the tension or pain by deep breathing.

Try this

○ Lie down on your bed. Become conscious of your breath. Sometimes counting can help you pay attention to your breathing. Notice your toes. Notice how they're feeling and try to relax them. Now notice your feet and relax them. Move gradually up your body, noticing each part. Don't rush. Try to do this slowly, relaxing each part of your body until you reach the top of your head. In addition to being a good relaxation technique, this exercise will help you notice each part of your body in your check-ins.

IN A SENTENCE:

> *Remember to make time for yourself. It's important to relax and reduce stress.*

Finding a Doctor Who's Right for You

"When I first found out I had hep C, my doctor knew very little about it. I realized I had to find a doctor who knew more. Fortunately, I had some friends with hep C, and one of them had just found a doctor who was really savvy. I went and saw him. We hit it off, and now I've been seeing him for the last three years. He's referred me to some really good specialists too."

—MIKE K.

DON'T SETTLE for a doctor you don't like. It's common for people just diagnosed with hep C to feel helpless and out of control. One of the most proactive and practical things you can do for yourself is to become an active patient and take charge of your health care. The first step is finding a hep C-aware doctor who's right for you. You may want to find more than one doctor or consult a specialist. If your doctor recommends anything drastic, you should get a second opinion.

We encourage you to interview several doctors and consider the following questions:

O Does this doctor accept your insurance?

O What is this doctor's expertise and background?

O Is the doctor affiliated with any universities, organizations, or studies? If so, which ones?

O Is the doctor available? Some doctors are so popular that you have to wait a long time for an appointment.

O How does your doctor treat you?

O Is the doctor able to explain research and treatments in a way that you can understand them?

O Will the doctor help you consider the pros and cons of every treatment you want to try?

O Do you prefer having a doctor who will let you have a lot of control in deciding your treatment options, or a doctor who will tell you what to do? If you like having a lot of control, it's a good idea to ask the doctor how he feels about that.

O Where is your doctor located? If you are fatigued, will you be able to get there?

O How does your doctor feel about supplements, herbs, acupuncture, and other alternative treatments? Does your doctor know anything about them? Is your doctor open to discussing them with you, or does he or she think they're all nonsense? If you've got your heart set on trying an alternative treatment, it's important to have a doctor who's at least open to talking with you about it and perhaps even doing some research.

You can search www.hep-c-alert.org to find a hep C–aware doctor in your area. Some other resources to help you find a hep C doctor are:

Hepatitis Directory of Online Resources:
www.objectivemedicine.com/dbsearch.htm

American Medical Associations Doctor Finder
webapps.ama-assn.org/doctorfinder/home.html

American Association of the Study of Liver Disease Physician Referral
www.aasld.org/eweb/StartPage.aspx?site=aasld3

If your insurance company is a health maintenance organization (HMO), it probably requires you to select a primary care provider (PCP) from its network. If you want to see another doctor, you have to get a referral from your PCP. It's important to select a PCP who knows something about hep C, or is at least willing to refer you to someone who specializes in your condition. The specialists you're likely to see include:

- A **gastroenterologist**, who specializes in disorders of the stomach and intestines, or
- A **hepatologist**, who specializes in the liver.

You may also want to see other health care professionals:

- A registered dietitian, if you need help coming up with a diet you can follow
- A physical therapist, to help you with your exercise plan, especially if you haven't exercised in a while or have limited mobility
- A mental health professional, to help you deal with any psychological issues around your diagnosis, such as depression.

In many cases, you can sign a disclosure form allowing your various doctors to talk to each other about your care. Nonetheless, it's unlikely that all the doctors you see in your life will talk to each other about the various treatments they're prescribing for you. It's important for you to keep medical records and keep each of your doctors informed. If your psychiatrist prescribes an antidepressant, for instance, make sure you tell your PCP about your new medication. Some drugs are hard on the liver. You may decide to take those drugs anyway, but if you do, it's a good idea to get your liver enzymes tested more frequently. A significant increase in your ALT and AST may indicate that the drug is damaging your liver. In 2000 Lisa went on the drug Accutane for acne. Since accutane can be damaging to the liver, she got her enzymes tested regularly. At first the drug didn't seem to be affecting them, but five months later they shot up, so she went off the drug.

In some cases, you may have difficulty finding a primary care physician or a doctor you can see on a consistent basis. When Lisa was diagnosed, her health insurance covered care at the university health clinic and occasionally authorized visits to specialists, but whenever she came into the clinic, she had to see a different doctor. There was a really fast turnover. People would work there for a half a year and then leave. The one good thing about this was that she learned to keep track of her own tests and get them every six months. In 1996 things got better, because more doctors at the clinic knew about hep C. She finally found a hep C–aware doctor she could see consistently.

IN A SENTENCE:

> *Find a doctor who is knowledgeable about hep C, and whom you can talk to.*

Diet: Eating for a Healthy Liver

"Hep C really got me in shape. I used to have a horrible diet. I ate all fried and processed foods. When I found out I had hep C, I decided to become a vegetarian. I had wanted to try this for years, and this was the final motivation. It was such a radical change for me. I lost 30 pounds, and I've never felt better in my life."

—JAMES W.

"I have cirrhosis, and my body can no longer break down fats as efficiently as it used to. The things I notice that affect me most are fatty foods and alcohol."

—KEVIN O.

DIETARY RECOMMENDATIONS for hep C patients vary widely. If you ask a nutritionist, a Chinese medical practitioner, and a conventional western doctor about diet, you might get very different advice from each.

Not everyone with hepatitis C needs to make drastic dietary changes. Chances are, you won't have to give up foods that you love forever. It's important that you find a diet that you can live with and practice on a consistent basis. A diet you can only follow for a few weeks won't do much good. Below we provide some basic guidelines on which foods may be harmful to your liver and which foods may be helpful. But diet, like any health program, is very individual. What works for one person might not work for another, and what works for you now may not work for the rest of your life, especially if the condition of your liver changes significantly. It's a good idea to see a dietician periodically to evaluate your diet and determine whether you should be changing your food choices.

> *"We talked about diet a lot in my support group. We would compare what worked for us and what didn't. Everyone was different. Some people said they had to avoid fried foods entirely, or they would get really sick. Other people said it didn't seem to make a difference."*
>
> —ALLEN S.

Foods that may place stress on the liver:

- Foods containing pesticides
- Foods containing added hormones. These include growth hormones that are fed to non-organically raised cows and chickens to make them grow faster and larger.
- Artificial flavors and colors, antibiotics and additives
- Fried foods, margarine and hydrogenated fats or "**trans-fats**," meaning any fat that is solid at room temperature.
- Sugar, which produces oxalic acid, which is hard for the liver to process
- Artificial sweeteners such as Nutrasweet™ and saccharine
- Meat, which produces nitrogeneous waste products, which are also hard on the liver.
- Dairy foods, such as milk, cheese, and ice cream. Yogurt is an exception because it is a probiotic—that is, a substance that promotes the growth of "good" bacteria, which boosts your immune system.

○ Raw or poorly cooked shellfish
○ Wild mushrooms
○ Shark cartilage
○ Foods high in iron, such as red meat. Excess iron hurts the liver, and HCV patients can't tolerate iron as well. Dark green leafy vegetables, such as raw spinach and collard greens, are also high in iron. However, these vegetables aren't much of a danger, because you probably won't overdose on iron from them, and they also provide vitamins and minerals your body needs. Just don't overdo it. Avoid cooking with iron cookware.
○ "Enriched" or "fortified" foods, like some cereals, are very high in iron. Half a cup of Kellogg's® Raisin Bran has as much iron as nine cups of spinach or three-quarters of a pound of steak. Dangerous.

Liver-friendly foods and beverages:

○ Water is one of the keys to detoxification. It helps things move through your body more easily. We've all been told to drink 8 glasses of water a day. With hep C this is even more important.
○ Carrots and carrot juice. Vitamin A in large doses is harmful. Getting vitamin A or beta carotene through carrots is much safer than taking a supplement.
○ Lean proteins
○ Dandelion greens, cabbage, asparagus, beets, garlic, onions, brussel sprouts, kale, mustard greens, turnip greens
○ High-fiber foods: fruits, vegetables, beans, and grains, such as brown rice, wheat, barley, oats, and rye
○ Soluble fiber, such as pectin, flax seed, guar gum, psyllium.

Many nutritionists recommend foods rich in **antioxidants**, such as the cabbage family, citrus, dandelion leaves, wheat germ, rosemary, yams, and winter squash, which contain vitamins A, C, and E. Our bodies naturally produce free radicals—highly reactive chemicals that mostly consist of toxic oxygen molecules. Just as oxygen can cause iron to rust, oxygen can corrode tissues such as blood vessel walls and liver cells. Oxidized liver cells are more susceptible to cirrhosis and cancer. Factors such as excess radiation, smoking, and a high-fat diet can multiply the number of free radicals, but foods rich in **antioxidants** can help reduce oxidative damage. The liver protects itself from oxidation by producing an enzyme called glutathione peroxidase. Large amounts of alcohol and Tylenol can damage the liver by interfering with the production of glutathione. Antioxidants such as vitamin E may prevent oxidation by boosting glutathione levels.[1]

There is controversy over whether people with hep C should take large amounts of vitamin C, because vitamin C will increase non-**heme** iron absorption. As we said above, too much iron is dangerous for people with hep C.

You can use the above lists as basic guidelines. If you're really invested in changing your diet, it's a good idea to consult a dietician or nutritionist. We are not medical doctors, and our suggestions in this chapter are no substitute for a doctor's advice. Be sure to check with your doctor before you embark on any new diet or exercise plan.

You may want to check out *The Hepatitis C Cookbook: Easy and Delicious Recipes* by Heather Jeanne (Cumberland House, 2004) or *A Real "Hep" Cookbook* by Ramona L. Jones, C.N.C., and Vonah L. Stanfield. You can order the latter from *Hepatitis* magazine. (*Liver Health Today* is the new name of this magazine.)

Hepatitis Magazine
523 N. Sam Houston Parkway East, Suite 300
Houston, TX 77060
281-272-2744 x133
www.hepatitismag.com

The Great Coffee Debate

IN THE LAST few decades, more than 19,000 scientific studies have examined coffee's effect on health. As it turns out, this much-maligned pick-me-up may reduce the risk of cirrhosis. A recent study, published in the *Archives of Internal Medicine*, followed more than 125,000 people for 15 to 22 years. The participants' likelihood of being diagnosed with alcoholic cirrhosis decreased approximately 22 percent with each cup of coffee they drank per day. Those who drank four or more cups per day had an 80 percent lower chance of developing alcoholic cirrhosis.[2] The study had some limitations, because the participants were only surveyed once, at the beginning of the study, on their alcohol, smoking, and coffee and tea drinking habits, and because researchers have no idea what ingredient in coffee is interacting with alcohol or protecting the liver. Lower rates of cirrhosis were not found among tea or decaf drinkers. Though this study did not find that coffee reduced the risk of nonalcoholic cirrhosis, several Italian studies reported an inverse relation between coffee consumption and cirrhosis in general: Subjects who drank three or more cups of coffee a day lessened their risk of cirrhosis by more than 70 percent.[3]

As with anything, it's important to weigh the advantages and disadvantages. Some of us feel that downing four or more javas a day would make us nervous wrecks. Physically active people have long been told to abstain from caffeinated drinks under the assumption that caffeine, a mild diuretic, will exacerbate the dehydration and electrolyte loss due to exercise. But scientific evidence may not back this up. A review of nine studies on this topic recently concluded, "The scientific literature suggests that athletes and recreational enthusiasts will not incur detrimental fluid-electrolyte imbalances if they consume caffeinated beverages in moderation and eat a typical U.S. diet."[4]

While we can't say coffee is the new health food, it seems to be a liver-friendly beverage, particularly for heavy drinkers. But don't think you can keep your liver happy by downing a pot of coffee after a bender. Experts say the best way to avoid alcoholic cirrhosis is, in fact, not to drink.

IN A SENTENCE:

Find a liver-friendly diet that works for you.

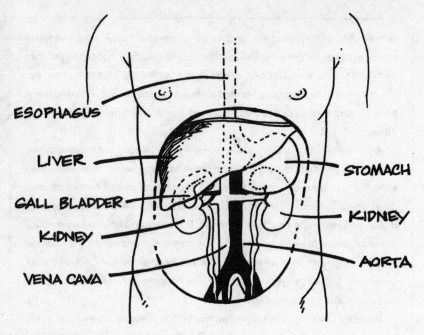

Location of the liver.

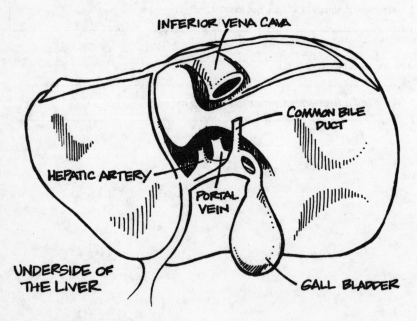

Underside of the liver.

Your Liver
and Its Functions

NOW THAT you have learned a bit about the virus, it will be helpful to know about the organ it primarily affects: the liver. Understanding your liver and how it works can help you take better care of it.

Your liver is your largest organ other than your skin. It weighs approximately 3 lbs. and is reddish-brown. Located on the right side of your abdomen beneath your diaphragm and behind your lower rib cage, it consists of four lobes of different sizes and shapes. It processes much of what you eat, drink, breathe, and absorb through your skin. Two major blood vessels carry oxygen and digested food to the liver. The hepatic artery brings oxygen-rich blood from the aorta, the largest artery in your body, to the liver. The portal vein picks up blood containing digested food from the small intestine and transports it to the liver.

Your liver performs many vital functions. It converts food into nutrients for energy and produces proteins, blood-clotting agents, and some immune factors.

○ Liver cells absorb carbohydrates, fats, and proteins.

○ The liver regulates the level of glucose in the blood. Liver cells transform glucose, a simple sugar, into glycogen, the form in which glucose is stored until the body needs it for energy.

○ In addition to storing sugar in the form of glycogen, the liver stores vitamins A, D, K, and B_{12} and minerals, such as iron.

○ The liver produces and secretes **bile**, which helps your body digest food and absorb nutrients. Bile, also called gall, contains water, bile pigments like bilirubin, bile acids and salts, fatty acids, and cholesterol. After the liver produces bile, the gall bladder acts as reservoir, storing bile and releasing it into the small intestine. Bile salts liquefy fats, so that they can be digested by the enzymes in the intestines.

○ After fats are broken down into fatty acids, the liver makes these fatty acids into cholesterol and other substances the body needs. The liver converts extra carbohydrates and protein into fat. It thus regulates the levels of fat and cholesterol.

○ As the liver breaks down protein, it produces the waste product urea. This process removes toxic ammonia from the body.

○ The liver regulates levels of chemicals and drugs in the blood. It metabolizes alcohol and removes toxins from the blood, discharging waste products into bile. Kupffer cells in the liver consume bacteria and waste products.

○ The liver makes some of the blood's necessary components, including plasma proteins and blood-clotting agents, such as prothrombin and fibrinogen.

○ The liver can make the nonessential amino acids.

○ It plays a function in maintaining hormonal balance.

○ It can also regenerate its own tissue. Three-fourths of the liver can be regenerated in a few weeks.

A diseased liver can affect the circulatory system, immune system, digestive system, brain, sex hormones, and kidneys. Since the liver processes much of what you eat, drink, breathe, and absorb through your skin, the best way to take care of your liver is to eat a healthy diet and avoid chemicals, including environmental pollutants, alcohol, and drugs, which are harmful to your liver.

IN A SENTENCE:

> *Your liver processes much of what you eat, drink, breathe, and absorb through your skin.*

living

Getting Exercise and Overcoming Insomnia

*"I was in a car accident and got hep C through a
blood transfusion. I have a lot of back pain from
the car accident. I have joint pain too. I don't
know if it's from my hep C or from the car
accident. Regardless of what it's from, I can't
exercise. I finally went to a physical therapist, who
got me started on a program. I go to the pool every
day and walk laps in the shallow end. I felt silly at
first, but the endorphins really kicked in, and my
pain has decreased. Now I notice when I don't
exercise for a day because I'm in more pain and
have more trouble sleeping."*

—LAURA K.

Finding an exercise program you can live with

THE SAME principles that apply to diet also apply to exercise: Namely, check with your doctor first, and find something

that you like to do and can live with. If you have physical limitations, such as joint pain, that make exercising more difficult, see a physical therapist who can figure out what kind of movement is best for you. Swimming is a low-impact exercise that's great for people who have joint pain or injuries.

A lot of people follow a new exercise regimen for a few weeks and then stop due to fatigue, boredom, or overcommitment. Some people find it easier to stick to their exercise plan when they exercise in the morning, simply because they run out of steam later in the day, or find that they have too many other things left to do.

It's hard to start a new exercise program, and it can be exhausting at first. But after the first six weeks you'll have more energy. Yoga and stretching can relieve muscle tension and reduce anxiety almost immediately. Aerobic exercise, which includes jogging, swimming, dancing, and fast walking, increases your heart rate and strengthens your cardiovascular system. Aerobic exercise also produces endorphins, which can alleviate depression and insomnia. This kind of exercise is especially helpful for anyone who is quitting an addiction to smoking, alcohol, or drugs. If you've just quit, it will take a few weeks before you can produce endorphins efficiently. But once the endorphins kick in, many recovering addicts say that they enjoy the high from exercise more than the high from their drug of choice.

Anaerobic exercise, such as weight lifting, strengthens your muscles and converts fat into muscle. If you want to start lifting weights, be sure to consult your doctor. Weight lifting can increase your blood pressure, so make sure you don't have any health problems that might be adversely affected. In general it's good to consult your doctor before embarking on any exercise plan, especially if you haven't exercised in a while, or if you're overweight, a smoker, or have high blood pressure or heart disease.

How to get started and keep exercising

- ○ If you have physical limitations, see a physical therapist, who can recommend an exercise plan for you.
- ○ Even if you don't have physical limitations, you might want to see a personal trainer, who can help you develop an exercise plan that's just right for you.

○ If you're extremely busy, find ways to fit exercise into your daily routine. Walk somewhere you need to go. Take the stairs instead of the elevator. Cara found she had no time to go to the gym. She invested in an exercise machine for her house, so she can work out whenever she has some extra time. Find something that works for you.

○ Make your exercise interesting. Take a walk with a friend. Find new places to explore on foot or bike around your home or work. When you visit a new city, explore it on foot.

○ Listen to music while you're walking, running, or using an exercise machine. It's also possible to read on some exercise machines. Lisa listens to her iPod while running on the beach and likes to read on the transport machines at the gym.

It's important that you warm up and cool down before and after each exercise session. If you are new to exercise, you might just want to start with walking. You can begin by walking at your usual pace for five minutes, then walk briskly for five minutes, and then walk normally again for five minutes. You can increase the amount of time that you walk briskly each day, until you are walking for an hour. When you walk briskly, try to reach your target heart rate.

Finding your target heart rate

The fastest way to achieve the maximum benefit from aerobic exercise is to reach your target heart rate range. However, any exercise that increases your pulse is helpful. Also, brief periods of exercise will provide aerobic benefit: It's not necessary to exercise for 20 to 30 minutes at a time. Exercise that makes your pulse faster than your target rate is not any better for your heart and lungs. To find your target heart rate range, subtract your age from 220 and multiply the result by two-thirds (0.67). This is the lower end of the target range. Three-quarters of 220 minus your age is the upper limit of your heart rate range.

How to take your pulse

○ Place the tip of your fingers on a pulse point, such as the one on your neck to the left or right of your Adam's apple or on your wrist below the bone of your thumb. Your doctor will be happy to show you how to take your pulse.

O Count the number of beats for a period of 30 seconds. Multiply that number by two to calculate how many times your heart is beating per minute.

Changes in sleep patterns: Stopping insomnia

"The worst part about having hep C is how much it messes with my sleep. Sometimes I am so fatigued, but I can't sleep. That drives me crazy. Someone in my support group told me to stop drinking coffee. I tried it, but it still doesn't help. My doctor won't give me sleep aids, because he's afraid they will hurt my liver. This is just one more losing battle for me."

—ERIC A.

Many people with hep C experience widely fluctuating sleep patterns. From debilitating fatigue to extreme insomnia, hepatitis C can wreak havoc on your circadian rhythms. Some people report night sweats, vivid or disturbing dreams, and the need to urinate frequently during the night. If you are experiencing insomnia, you may want to try to stop drinking caffeine, especially within 8 hours of your bedtime. While this may seem impossible if you are tired much of the time, it will most likely help you sleep better. Aerobic exercise and stress reduction can also relieve insomnia. Cara suffers from difficulty sleeping and has found that Dr. Zhang's sleep formula *Herbsom* helps her. You can find Dr. Zhang's herbal preparations at www.dr-zhang.com/home.htm. As always, be sure to consult your doctor before you begin taking herbs, or if you experience extreme insomnia.

Here are some tips for alleviating insomnia:

O Start "unwinding" an hour before bedtime.
O Make your sleeping environment more comfortable. Adjust the temperature. Buy softer sheets if necessary.
O Use your bed only for sleeping, not for watching TV, reading, or eating. (This way, you'll have a Pavlovian response: you'll go to sleep when you get into bed, just like those dogs who salivate at the sound of a bell that always rings before mealtime.)

○ If you don't fall asleep within 20 minutes, get out of bed and do something relaxing until you feel tired again. Keep the lights dim and the TV and computer off.

○ Avoid eating within three hours of your bedtime.

○ Avoid sitting under bright lights, watching TV, and using the computer before bedtime.

○ Don't watch horror movies before bed.

○ Wake up at the same time every day, regardless of how long you sleep.

○ Keep a log of the time you go to bed, how long it takes you to fall asleep, and the time you wake up. Keeping a record of an activity such as sleep will help you become more conscious of your habits, and this is often half the battle in alleviating the problem.

○ Limit your naps to 20 to 30 minutes in the early afternoon. Napping at night or taking two- or three-hour naps during the day can make you less sleepy at bedtime.

○ Drink warm milk (which contains tryptophan) or chamomile tea to make yourself drowsy.

○ Give up or cut back on caffeine, nicotine, and alcohol.

○ It's important to drink lots of water, but if you wake up frequently with a full bladder, you might want to stop drinking fluids two or three hours before bedtime.

○ If insomnia continues, seek a doctor's help, and consider possible causes such as sleep apnea. Selective seratonin reuptake inhibitors (SSRIs) can help with sleep disturbances—especially those related to depression or anxiety.

It's important for people with hep C to avoid relying on alcohol or sleeping pills as sedatives. Some herbs, such as kava and valerian, can cause severe liver damage in people without hepatitis and should be avoided.

IN A SENTENCE:

A good exercise program can improve your overall health, help you get in shape, reduce stress, and regulate your sleep patterns.

learning

The Effects of Different Drugs on the Liver

Drugs and liver disease

I was on an anti-anxiety drug for ten years. I just found out that seven-eighths of my liver is cirrhotic. Apparently I had hep C all along and my liver disease progressed really fast.

—JAMES E.

AS WE discussed in the last chapter, your liver processes most of what you eat, drink, breathe, and absorb through your skin. Since hepatitis C already places stress on your liver, it's a good idea to reduce your intake of substances that can accelerate liver damage. In Day 2, we discussed the importance of avoiding alcohol. In the following section, we elaborate on some pharmaceutical and recreational drugs that may be toxic to the liver.

There are many ways drugs can damage the liver. Some drugs hurt the liver directly. In other cases, the drug itself is not harmful, but as the liver processes the substance, it produces by-products that kill liver cells. The three major types of drug-induced liver toxicity are dose-dependent, idiosyncratic, and drug allergy. While these kinds of toxicity can affect anyone, it is important for people with hepatitis C to be especially cautious.

Dose-dependent toxicity means that the drug may cause liver damage if you take more than a certain amount. One example is acetaminophen (Tylenol). When the liver metabolizes acetaminophen, it produces some potentially toxic metabolites (or byproducts). A chemical called glutathione binds to these metabolites and prevents them from harming the liver. This system works fine, as long as a person takes the recommended dosage of Tylenol. When a person takes more than 15 grams of Tylenol at once, the liver runs out of glutathione, leaving the metabolites free to cause liver damage. This is how Tylenol poisoning occurs. A healthy adult should ingest no more than four doses (two g) per day for a maximum of 10 days and avoid alcohol. Children should not take Tylenol for more than five days, and people with liver dysfunction should ask their doctors for advice.

Idiosyncratic toxicity occurs when a person has inherited a specific gene that prevents her liver from processing the drug the way others do, and the drug or its metabolites build up and harm her liver. This type of toxicity is rare and usually emerges only after a drug is FDA-approved and millions are taking it. Some drugs are more prone to being idiosyncratic than others. Liver disease from drug allergy is also uncommon. A drug allergy causes the immune system to attack the drug with antibodies, and the resulting inflammation harms the liver.

As we discussed, people with hep C should have their liver enzymes (ALT and AST) checked every three months. If you have to take a drug that can cause liver damage, your doctor may want to monitor your liver enzymes more frequently, and you may have to discontinue the drug if your ALT and AST rise dramatically. If your liver enzymes are already elevated due to hepatitis C, it can be especially difficult for doctors to determine whether you have a drug-induced toxicity. Be aware of any new symptoms or exacerbations of old ones, such as fatigue. Jaundice is not a common symptom of hep C, so if your skin or the whites of your eyes turn yellow, contact your doctor immediately.

Here's a list of medications that can be toxic to your liver.

O   anabolic steroids
O   corticosteroids (prednisone)

O acetaminophen (Tylenol). (As indicated above, this is safe when taken as recommended and not combined with alcohol. Note: Infant acetaminophen suspension drops are far more concentrated than the medicine for children. Don't give a baby more than a dropperful of infant Tylenol. If you give the baby a teaspoon, it can be poisonous.)
O NSAIDs (aspirin, naproxen)
O ibuprofen
O barbiturates
O benzodiazepines, especially Halcion, but also diazepam (Valium), Xanax, Klonopin, etc.
O some antidepressants, such as amitriptyline
O chlorpromazine (Thorazine)
O bactrim
O birth control pills
O haldol
O some antibiotics, including ciprofloxin, clindamycin (Cleocin), erythromycin estolate, tetracycline, metronidazole (Flagyl), amoxicillin
O pemoline (Cylert)
O phenytoin (Dilantin)
O cimetidine (Tagamet)
O statins (cholesterol-reducing medications)

This list is not exhaustive and does not substitute for a doctor's advice. Ask your doctor before taking any medication. Even drugs that are relatively safe when taken alone can be dangerous when combined with other drugs, so it is important to inform your doctor of all medications you're taking, as well as vitamins and supplements. Of course, it's never a bad idea to educate yourself. Doctors aren't infallible. They sometimes have a hard time keeping track of all the medications their patients are taking, especially those prescribed by other doctors.

The Drug Induced Liver Injury Network is a great place to check if a medication you are taking is harmful to your liver.

http://dilin.dcri.duke.edu/

We also look up the precautions and interactions of various drugs on MEDLINEplus, a source of accurate, up-to-date information provided by the National Library of Medicine at the National Institutes of Health (NIH). The URL is www.nlm.nih.gov/medlineplus/. When you look up a drug, look under the sections entitled "Precautions for Using this Medicine."

MEDLINEplus can provide information about various health conditions and diseases. The site also contains links to multilingual medical dictionaries, various hospitals, doctors, and clinical trials. We'll talk more about MEDLINE and MEDLINEplus in Month 7, "Keeping Up-to-Date and Doing Research."

Valium, Xanax, and other benzodiazepines

Benzodiazepines (Valium, Xanax, Klonopin, etc.) are popular prescription drugs, but they can be especially dangerous for people with liver dysfunction and older people. The liver mainly processes medications and other substances through two processes: oxidation and conjugation. These account for more than 90 percent of the liver's reactions. Benzodiazepines are both conjugated and oxidized. In hepatic dysfunction and aging, the liver can lose the ability to oxidize, which means that the person cannot metabolize the drug and can overdose more easily. Studies have also shown that benzos can worsen hepatitis. For these reasons, most doctors avoid prescribing benzos to HCV-positive patients. Lorazepam (Ativan), oxazepam (Serax) and temazepam (Restoril) are the safest, because they are mostly conjugated rather than oxidized, but even these should be avoided. If a patient with a compromised liver needs to take a benzo, her doctor will usually lower the dosage to about one-half or one-fourth of the regular dose and watch for signs of overdose, such as dizziness, blurred vision, slurred speech, and excessive sedation.

Medical marijuana

Medical cannabis is less toxic than many pharmaceutical preparations, and it can be used to treat some symptoms of hep C, including loss of appetite, insomnia, and slight joint pain. A few studies have indicated that smoking marijuana may be carcinogenic, but these results are still controversial. Some regular cannabis smokers report more frequent lung and throat infections and decreased lung capacity. If you are concerned, inhaling cannabis through a vaporizer is probably safer and less irritating to the throat and lungs than smoking it in a joint, pipe, or bong.[1]

Laws regarding the use of medical marijuana vary widely from state to state. These laws are constantly in flux, and they are not always recognized by local law enforcement agencies. In California, for instance, it is legal to take medical marijuana with your doctor's permission, but in practice, local law enforcement may crack down on you for the use of cannabis. Thus, it's wise to familiarize yourself with the laws and law enforcement patterns in your area before using marijuana for medical purposes. You can contact the following organizations for up-to-date information:

Marijuana Policy Project
P.O. Box 77492
Capitol Hill
Washington, D.C. 20013
202-462-5747
www.mpp.org

Americans for Medical Rights
1250 Sixth Street, #202
Santa Monica, CA 90401
310-394-2952
Fax: 310-451-7494
www.medmjscience.org
www.drugreform.org

Smoking tobacco

Many people give up alcohol and other drugs before they give up smoking. There are at least two good reasons to do this:

O Drugs and alcohol addictions can be far more dangerous and detrimental to your overall life.
O It's often easier to quit smoking when you're no longer drinking and doing drugs.

Nonetheless, the health hazards of smoking are well documented, and smoking can be particularly dangerous for people with compromised livers or immune systems.

○ Smoking can increase one's susceptibility to liver damage from potentially hepatotoxic medications.
○ Smoking can impair the liver's ability to detoxify hazardous substances, including the toxins in cigarettes.
○ Severe liver damage can impede blood circulation, and smoking can exacerbate this problem.
○ Although smoking is more often associated with lung and throat cancer, those of us with hep C have a higher risk of liver cancer, and smoking may increase this risk.

Recreational drugs

In Day 2 we referred to alcohol as the liver's number one enemy. Recreational drugs can also be dangerous. Even if the drug itself is not toxic to the liver, street drugs are almost always "cut" or diluted with other substances to increase profits. The "cut"—which can be anything from sugar to caffeine to toilet bowl cleaner to rat poison—may be far more hazardous to your health than the drug. Consequently, it is never a good idea to be the first person to try a drug you've bought from a stranger on the street. If you do drugs, practice the harm reduction strategy that kings and emperors have used for centuries: have a taste-tester sample your food before you eat it. This does not mean you should poison your friends. Just make a commitment to yourself that you will only take drugs from a trusted source or from a batch that others have taken.

In this section we provide some information on the relative toxicity of various drugs and some harm reduction guidelines. Keep in mind that it is hard to study the long-term effects of different recreational drugs, because most drug users don't know what their drugs are cut with. Researchers can give a cohort of people methamphetamine and study its effects, but a group of long-term speed users who bought their drugs on the street will have taken very different combinations of substances, even if they say they "only used crystal meth."

Stimulants

Many stimulants are relatively safe when used for medical purposes. This is true of medications such as methylphenidate (Ritalin), dexmethylphenidate

(Focalin), dextroamphetamine (Dexedrine), and dextroamphetamine combined with racemic salts (Adderall), which are used to treat attention deficit disorder, narcolepsy, and chronic fatigue. When used recreationally, amphetamine (speed), methamphetamin (crystal meth), and cocaine are hard on the body—causing sleeplessness and immune suppression. Cocaine can cause acute hepatitis. Other stimulants can also lead to liver disease, especially with prolonged use and when combined with alcohol.

It's best for people with hep C to avoid recreational stimulants. If you do use them, you can take the following steps for harm reduction:

○ Cut back on the amount and frequency you use, and give yourself plenty of time to recover. Don't keep yourself awake for days or weeks.
○ Drink lots of water.
○ Avoid alcohol. (This is especially important. Many people on coke or speed drink in order to relax or "come down." They may also drink more than usual because the stimulant counteracts alcohol's sedative effects, so they get drunk less quickly.)
○ If you shoot up, don't share any works or reuse equipment. Remember that bleach may not kill the hep C virus. If you do have to reuse, the safest way to disinfect is full immersion for at least 20 minutes in full strength bleach.

MDMA (Ecstasy)

MDMA has gained lots of media attention for its potential as a neurotoxin, but it might also cause liver damage. It is relatively rare for people on Ecstasy to require emergency medical services, but 16 percent of reported medical problems are liver-related. Many of these problems are associated with hyperthermia. Most MDMA-related deaths are due to heatstroke: someone on "E" is dancing at a rave and collapses. It is well documented that hyperthermia can cause liver damage. Several in vitro studies have indicated that MDMA can damage liver cells at normal body temperature, but overheating increases the risk.[2]

Tips for harm reduction:

○ Get the Ecstasy tested for purity.
○ Drink lots of water.

○ Don't overexert yourself by dancing all night or doing some other strenuous activity that could lead to overheating. (You'll be less inclined to do this if your Ecstasy is not cut with speed.)
○ Avoid drinking alcohol while on Ecstasy.

LSD

LSD (acid) is not directly hepatotoxic, but it is hard on the entire body because its effects can last 12 hours or more. A lot of acid is cut with speed, which can keep you awake for days. If you take acid, you can practice harm reduction by taking pure LSD, drinking lots of water, getting enough sleep and avoiding alcohol.

Magic mushrooms

Hallucinogenic mushrooms containing psilocybin and psilocin are not hepatotoxic. When someone dies from mushroom poisoning, it is usually because they have mistaken a poisonous mushroom for a safe one. Most poisonous mushrooms contain amatoxins and come from the genera Amanita, Galerina, Lepiota, and Conocybe. Amatoxin poisoning can cause death in seven to ten days due to liver failure.[3]

Opioids

Many drugs fall under the category of opiates. Opiates are narcotic analgesics used in the treatment of pain. The opiate family includes morphine, heroin, methadone, buprenorphine, codeine, Oxycodone, alfentanil, fentanyl, meperidine (Demerol), remifentanil, and tramadol (Ultram). The majority of opiates are not harmful to your liver. But OxyContin, Percocet, Darvocet, and Vicodin all contain acetaminophen, which makes them dangerous to the liver if taken in large amounts. Heroin itself is not particularly dangerous to the liver in its pure form, but if you buy it on the street it will be cut with something, and that additive could be very dangerous. Also, a drug-using lifestyle—which often includes lack of proper nutrition, sleep, and exercise and the abuse of other drugs—can strain the liver.

If you have liver dysfunction, some opiates may not work or may lead to an unintentional overdose. Morphine and meperidine must be used with special care to avoid overdose. Dextropropoxyphene can be hepatoxic to an already decompensated liver and should be avoided. Cirrhotic patients may also lose the ability to metabolize codeine and tramadol, so other painkillers should be prescribed instead.

A few studies indicate that morphine use and withdrawal may be particularly harmful for people with hep C and for those undergoing interferon-based treatments. As we discuss below in Week 4, our immune cells produce antiviral proteins called **interferons**, which "interfere" with viral replication. Part of the standard therapy for patients with hep C is a synthetic interferon, modeled on the natural interferons our body produces. A recent study has found that morphine enhances hepatitis C viral replication and inhibits the production of natural interferon. Morphine may also decrease the effectiveness of the synthetic interferons used for treating hep C patients. Another study has found that morphine withdrawal can impede interferon production in the liver, thus making the liver a better environment for HCV. Consequently, patients dependent on morphine are advised to go on methadone maintenance or bupenorphine.[4]

Drugs that help you get off recreational drugs

METHADONE

Methadone is the oldest and most common "substitution treatment" for opiate dependency. It's a synthetic opioid that alleviates withdrawal symptoms and cravings for opiates. Methadone undergoes oxidative biotransformation in the liver, but is also stored in the liver and released into the blood in unchanged form. It can be used in patients with chronic liver disease and advanced cirrhosis, but in acute liver disease or decompensated cirrhosis, patients must be monitored for signs of narcotic overdose or withdrawal symptoms. In these cases, the methadone dose must be lowered.

Ninety percent of people on methadone have hepatitis C. A research study by University of California at San Francisco and the Organization to Achieve Solutions in Substance-Abuse (O.A.S.I.S.) found that methadone-maintenance patients on interferon-based therapy had similar response rates to non-IDU patients. They recommend that methadone maintenance patients be considered for HCV treatment. Another study, by Stefan Mauss, reported data from 100 HCV-positive subjects: 50 were on methadone maintenance for at least six months, and 50 had not used street drugs or any substitution treatment for at least five years. Approximately 60 percent had genotype 1, and all received the current standard treatment of Peg-Intron plus ribavirin. At the end of the study the methadone maintenance group had a 42 percent sustained response rate, compared to 56 percent in the nonuser group. The researchers concluded that the standard HCV treatment is safe and effective to give to patients on methadone maintenance.

Treatment for hep C is becoming more inclusive. More clinical trials are accepting patients on methadone and bupenorphine. The National Institutes of Health (NIH) now states that treatment should be made available to patients previously considered untreatable: drug users, the mentally ill, prisoners, and participants in methadone maintenance programs.

Find a methadone clinic near you: http://www.treatmentfinder.com/?geo.

BUPENORPHINE

Like methadone, bupenorphine is a substitute for heroin, morphine, oxycodone, and other opiates. Buprenorphine, a derivative of the morphine alkaloid thebaine, is a partial opioid agonist working at the micro opioid receptor in the nervous system. Like methadone, buprenorphine is legal and can help IV drug users stop shooting up and thus prevent the spread of viruses such as HCV, HIV, and HBV. While methadone users have to go to a clinic to get their medication, a doctor with a special license can write a prescription for bupenorphine, so a patient can take this medication in the privacy of his own home. Many people claim they have far fewer withdrawal symptoms with bupenorphine than with methadone. A partial opiate, bupenorphine doesn't make you feel as "high" as methadone, but it does take away the craving for heroin and often for cocaine. Bupenorphine can come with or without naloxone, an opiate blocker, which will keep you from getting high—a good deterrent if you need it. It also has a long half-life, enabling you to go longer between doses if necessary.

Bupenorphine is mostly safe for people with hepatitis C. It has been used to treat opiate dependency in France since 1987 with very few hepatotoxic results. There have, however, been a few cases of bupenorphine-induced hepatitis, especially when users have injected the medication. Even when taken the proper sublingual way, there have been rare cases of liver dysfunction. Doctors must monitor liver functions closely in HCV patients on bupenorphine, and it is extremely important not to inject this drug.

Neither bupenorphine nor methadone has been shown to influence the effects of interferon and ribavirin during hepatitis C treatment. While many clinical trials still exclude any former or active substance abusers, others are now opening their doors to people who have been stable on bupenorphine for at least six months.[5]

To find a doctor who can prescribe bupenorphine near you: www.buprenorphine.samhsa.gov/.

IN A SENTENCE:

> *Smoking, some recreational drugs, and some medications can be toxic to the liver.*

FIRST-WEEK MILESTONE

By the end of your first week, you've learned the basic information about hep C and made the changes you can make immediately:

- ○ YOU'VE MADE TIME FOR YOURSELF TO DEAL WITH THE SHOCK OF YOUR DIAGNOSIS.

- ○ YOU'VE LEARNED THE BASIC INFORMATION ABOUT HEP C AND HOW IT IS TRANSMITTED.

- ○ YOU'VE GOTTEN YOUR FIRST VACCINATIONS FOR HEP A AND HEP B, OR AT LEAST MADE APPOINTMENTS TO GET THEM.

- ○ YOU'VE TALKED WITH PEOPLE WHO NEED TO KNOW IMMEDIATELY ABOUT YOUR DIAGNOSIS.

- ○ YOU'VE LEARNED ABOUT LIVER-FRIENDLY DIETS AND BEGUN TO MAKE DIET AND EXERCISE CHANGES.

- ○ YOU'VE LEARNED WHAT TESTS YOU NEED AND HOW TO READ THE RESULTS.

- ○ YOU'VE BEGUN TO LOOK FOR A HEP C–AWARE DOCTOR WHO'S RIGHT FOR YOU.

Prioritizing Lifestyle Changes

*"The beauty of hep C is that it gets you healthy.
Literally. Whatever junk-scarfing, dope-taking, ho-
bagging kind of freak you were before you got the
news, step into a room with some well-coiffed MD
who tells you that, thanks to your racy lifestyle, you
could be dead in a year—depending on whether your
liver goes straight into full-on cirrhosis and cancer
mode, or takes its time about it—and the words
'wake-up call' don't get within shouting distance of
conveying the frisson of mortality that screams from
your spinal cord to your scrotum and back up again.
This is Uh-Oh Time, plain and simple. And, in my
case, at least, it's made for a life of weirdly
intoxicating wholesomeness. Having been a dope
fiend of one kind or another from teen-hood to the
tail end of my thirties, I—like so many human waste
dumps of my acquaintance—have basically been old
already. So, despite the bad liver—or because of it—
I have adopted a life heavily involved with gyms and
yoga, running and Qi Gong, wheatgrass and milk*

*thistle, nonconsumption of alcohol, happy pills, or coffee.
Reading this, it does sound a little revolting, but trust me,
straight reality is The Last Frontier. The truly peculiar effect of
all the above is that, having been diagnosed with a potentially
terminal disease, I have never felt healthier. Junkies who've
made it out of junk tend to actually look and feel okay. My
theory is that we got a lot of rest, but who knows? The point is,
I've been old already. I was sick for years. But now I'm not sick,
I'm just dying. And I've never felt better.
Except when I feel like shit."*

—JERRY STAHL

AS PEOPLE with hep C, we can keep our livers a lot healthier by
avoiding drugs and alcohol. As we mentioned above, even a moderate consumption of alcohol greatly increases our chances of progressing toward cirrhosis. The consumption of other drugs may increase these chances as
well. For some of us, drugs will be a minor issue or not an issue at all. But
many of us are facing serious drug and alcohol addictions. If you have an
addiction, quitting it is most likely the most important thing you can do to
live a healthy life with hep C. It will be difficult to make positive changes
in your life until you take care of the addiction.

Answer the questions below in your journal:

○ What is the one thing that is most important for you to change?
○ What do you feel that you most want to change?
○ Note any resistances surrounding these changes. Write about the
feelings that come up for you.

Tips for breaking addictions or reducing harm

If you are struggling with an addiction, we strongly recommend you talk
to a doctor or addiction specialist, such as a counselor at a methadone
clinic or detox center, because withdrawal symptoms from some drugs can
be dangerous.

○ Decide what you need to quit first. As we said above, it's better to
eliminate substances one at a time. You have a better chance of

quitting alcohol, for instance, if you don't try to stop smoking at the same time. Ask yourself the following questions:

O What's most harmful to your liver?

O What's most damaging to your overall life? For instance, heroin may be less toxic to the liver than some other drugs, but the heroin lifestyle may be much more damaging and dangerous.

O If you can, go to a rehab center. That's one of the most effective ways to quit, but many people don't have the time or the money. If you can't go to a rehab center, try to get some other help—like the support of professionals and/or friends. Realize that you don't have to do it alone. People who quit in group settings are more likely to stay clean. Check out your local 12-step program or find something equivalent. Many people go to 12-step programs or Harm Reduction Programs. There are 12-step programs for people of many spiritual persuasions. If you find that you can't get clean right away, Harm Reduction Programs teach you how you can reduce harm to your liver and keep yourself safer and healthier.

O Realize that even if you're not quitting cold turkey but just reducing your consumption, you may experience some symptoms of withdrawal. It's a good idea to get professional help, because withdrawal from some substances can be dangerous. The symptoms of withdrawal from alcohol and benzodiazepines can include seizures, delirium tremens, and even death. Get information on what the detox might involve. It's extremely important to get the help of a support group or therapist as well as a medical professional, because when you withdraw from drugs or alcohol, all the feelings the substance has been repressing come rushing back.

One of the most damaging philosophies in our society is that quitting a drug addiction is nearly impossible. Many people stop an addiction each year. It can be done. Positive thinking and having faith in yourself are two of your strongest allies. Even if you experience some relapses, don't beat yourself up. The most important thing to do is get back on your feet and try again. You can do it.

Develop a concrete schedule for your lifestyle changes. Then come up with a timeline for putting this plan in action.

○ If you are not ready to stop using immediately, or if you are not going to stop using everything at once, keep a record of your drug and alcohol consumption. This can help you get a realistic view of how much you are actually using.

○ Write down realistic goals. Don't try to quit everything at once. For example, if you are quitting heroin, don't worry about quitting smoking at the same time.

○ Make a schedule for quitting and begin getting the appropriate help.

○ Post your schedule somewhere where you'll see it enough to keep it in the front of your mind.

○ Keep track of your detox schedule. Often it's helpful to mark the days you don't use with stickers or something on a calendar so you can easily chart your progress. Twelve-step programs reward people for time in the program by giving them chips.

○ Make an exercise schedule that goes hand in hand with your detox schedule. People who exercise regularly are statistically more likely to stay clean. Producing natural endorphins through exercise helps relieve withdrawal symptoms and cravings.

Changing a lifestyle can be difficult, but it is our experience that when we take action to change the aspects of our lifestyle and health that we can control, the things we can't control seem lighter. Taking care of the future frees us up to live in the present.

"I had to get clean because I was going to die. I was so sick with hepatitis. I just kept getting sicker and sicker, and I still couldn't stop doing dope. Finally I checked myself into a psych ward because I knew that the only way I was going to stop doing dope was if I was locked up."

—TRISH S.

"When I found out that I had hep C, it was a big reality check. I had been using IV drugs for years, and this was the first real consequence of my actions. Getting hep C made me realize that I was hurting myself and ruining my life. It made me want to stop."

—JOE T.

"I gave up heroin three years ago. I still get cravings. I go to NA meetings every day, sometimes twice a day, and that helps."

—KELLY D.

"I was doing a lot of drugs, drinking and smoking when I found out I had hep C. I know a lot of people on the streets who have hep C and just don't care. They don't even care if they die. I freaked out and tried to stop everything at once, cold turkey, but totally relapsed. I went to the methadone clinic, and somebody talked to me about harm reduction. We made a schedule for me to quit everything one at a time and slowly. I gave up the heroin and alcohol first and got on methadone. I still smoke, and I'm still on methadone. I'm also staying away from all my friends who shoot up. I avoid needles like the plague."

—JENNY R.

"Twelve-step programs didn't work for me. I had to go to rehab and be watched 24 hours a day. That was the only way it was going to work for me. Now I go to the 12-step programs, but they only worked for me after my month in rehab."

—TODD B.

IN A SENTENCE:

> *Reducing alcohol and drug intake as much as possible may be the most important step you can take to keep your liver healthy.*

learning

Insurance and Financial Planning

*"I work for a small company. I went on interferon,
which is an expensive medication, and people
are pissed that they have to pay higher
insurance premiums."*

—BOB J.

Why you need insurance

WHEN YOU have a chronic condition, you have to plan for a lifetime of health care expenses. There's no question that you will have costly medical bills, and you'll need insurance to cover them. This can be a huge cause of anxiety, especially if you don't have insurance when you're diagnosed, or if you're already sick and immediately have to deal with major expenses.

Even if you're healthy for years, you'll still have to get regular checkups and lab tests to monitor your enzymes and liver functions. In the best-case scenario, you'll have to pay for liver panels every six months and annual exams. If you pursue the drug therapy that is currently most effective—pegylated interferon in combination with ribavirin—48 weeks of medication may cost as much as $30,000, not including doctors' visits, blood work, and other tests you might need. Not all insurance covers interferon treatment. Liver transplants cost an average of $250,000. Fortunately more and more insurance companies are covering transplants, but a lifetime of immunosuppressive drugs is a huge out-of-pocket expense, if your insurance doesn't cover it. Alternative treatments, such as acupuncture, are usually less expensive than conventional western procedures, but your insurance is less likely to pay for them.

This section provides an introduction to the subject of health insurance, but you need to do some research on your own, since laws change and vary from state to state. At the end of each section, we provide resources to help you do more in-depth research. The information and suggestions in this chapter are all subject to change and are no substitute for a doctor or lawyer's advice. It's also advisable to talk to a number of different insurance companies before you decide on a plan.

If you already have insurance

If you already have insurance when you're diagnosed, you're fortunate. Your insurance can't kick you off of its plan just because you now have a chronic illness. Find out what your plan covers. Read your policy. If your insurance refuses to cover something, be persistent—or ask your doctor to be persistent. You or your doctor may have to request coverage—of a prescription drug, for instance—several times before your insurance agrees to pay for it. Remember that your insurance company is interested in saving money in the long run. One way to persuade an insurance company to cover a relatively low medical bill is to provide evidence that you are doing everything you can to prevent the need for much more costly treatments in the future. Chances are, your insurance company would rather pay for routine blood work, a liver biopsy, or substance abuse counseling than pay for a liver transplant 20 years from now.

If you leave your job

Government legislation allows someone to take her group health insurance policy when leaving employment or changing jobs. COBRA has strict time limits. For example, you have 60 days to enroll in COBRA after leaving your job. You then have 45 days to pay your premium. You may only keep COBRA for 18 months. If you become disabled, you may keep COBRA for 29 months. If you become divorced or separated, you may keep it for 36 months. Check out:

www.cobrahealth.com
www.dol.gov/dol/topic/health-plans/cobra.htm
www.dol.gov/ebsa/faqs/faq_consumer_cobra.html

If you change jobs

Before you change jobs, find out what health benefits you'll receive at your new job. Make sure the new insurance will cover hep C, even though you were diagnosed with it while you were still at your old job. Make sure you weigh all your options. Don't stay in a job you hate just because it offers good health benefits, and don't turn down a huge raise just because you'll lose a relatively small amount of health insurance.

Applying for insurance with a preexisting condition

Unfortunately, it's hard to get insurance if you've already been diagnosed with hep C. If you've ever filled out an insurance application, you've probably had to answer a series of questions about whether you've ever been diagnosed with various medical conditions. A preexisting condition is a condition that you were diagnosed with before you applied for the insurance. Insurance companies usually turn down people with preexisting conditions, such as hepatitis C, HIV, asthma, diabetes, and cancer, because they know that these people will have costly medical bills. Thus most insurance companies will deny you coverage if you've tested positive for HCV. If you're at risk for hep C but don't have insurance, it's wise to be tested anonymously or wait until you have insurance before you get tested.

Fortunately, if you have a preexisting condition and your job doesn't provide health benefits, it's not the end of the world. You can still join some sort of group or union to get on its group plan. There are lots of groups that writers, actors, dancers, and other self-employed people can join in order to get insurance coverage. Their group rates are lower than individual premiums.

If your employer provides medical benefits, you don't have to worry as much about preexisting conditions. Nonetheless, it's important to know your company's policies for dealing with disability, including sick days and short-term disability leave. Some companies require that a doctor of their choice evaluate whether or not you're capable of working.

○ Keep copies of all your medical records, just in case you ever have to prove that you can't work.

○ If you're feeling sick, be sure to keep a daily journal of your symptoms and how they interfere with your ability to perform daily tasks.

○ Tell your friends about the difficulties you're having, in case you ever need to apply for government health insurance. Government forms require family and friends to describe how your illness affects your daily life.

Guaranteed issue

Some states require all insurance companies to offer at least a few health insurance plans to people with preexisting conditions without a waiting period. Each state has its own requirements, so you should contact your state's Department of Insurance. For contact information for each state:

www.ican2000.com/state.html.

Open enrollment

Some states require Blue Cross/Blue Shield to open their enrollment at least once a year to anyone who applies for health insurance, regardless of preexisting conditions or medical history. To find out if your state offers this, call your local Blue Cross/Blue Shield and ask about their "open enrollment for individual health plans."

www.bcbs.com/

HIPAA (Health Insurance Portability Accountability Act)

Passed by Congress in 1996, the Health Insurance Portability Accountability Act protects the electronic transmission of medical records and makes it easier for people with preexisting conditions to change jobs without losing their health insurance. It also helps people obtain individual health insurance when they lose group health insurance and prevents health insurance plans from discriminating against people with medical conditions. When you switch from a group to an individual policy you must meet certain criteria. You must have been covered by the group insurance for 18 months without a 63-day lapse in coverage, and you must have elected and exhausted COBRA coverage. States that do not elect HIPAA must offer an alternative major medical policy. This is usually a high-risk pool.

You can find information on HIPAA here: www.dol.gov/dol/topic/health-plans/portability.htm.

High-risk pools

A high-risk pool is usually a state-created, sometimes nonprofit, association that offers health insurance benefits to people with preexisting conditions. Currently, 32 states offer a high-risk alternative. Each program has its own strict eligibility requirements, but most are open to people who have been denied coverage in the past because they have a chronic illness or a high-cost medical condition, or because they only qualify for restricted coverage.

The major problem high-risk pools face is funding. Critics have pointed out that few people actually enroll in high-risk pools, but others say that the high-risk pools are meeting the needs of the targeted population. Many people don't know about high-risk pools and don't know if they are eligible. The State Coverage Initiatives site (statecoverage.net/matrix/high riskpools.htm) has a list of all states that offer high-risk insurance.

For contact information for each state: www.ican2000.com/state.html

> *"My girlfriend found out that she had hep C.*
> *We had been doing IV drugs together, so I was pretty sure*
> *that I had it too. But I don't have insurance, and I don't want*
> *to get tested before I have insurance, because then I will have*
> *a preexisting condition and won't be able to get insurance."*
>
> —MARK O.

"I wish I had gotten an anonymous hep C test. Now I have this on my record, and there is nothing I can do about it."

—KATE H.

The cost of chronic conditions

Seven out of 10 deaths in the U.S. are attributed to chronic illness. Yet, less than 10 percent of each state's health department budget is allocated toward preventing chronic disease. The number of people with chronic conditions is growing fast. According to Partnership for Solutions, by the year 2020, 25 percent of U.S. citizens will be living with multiple chronic conditions. The United States currently spends one trillion dollars on health care each year. Sixty percent of this goes toward caring for the chronically ill. By 2020, the cost for managing chronic conditions alone will reach $1.07 trillion.

Disease management

Many people suffering from chronic conditions face outrageous medical bills, unemployment, and trouble navigating the health care and medical insurance systems. A new movement called disease management may be the key for people living with chronic illness. Disease management companies will coordinate all the long-term care a person needs. People with chronic illnesses are living longer and require more help and care throughout their lifetimes. More young people are suffering from chronic conditions and can live for decades with a disease. All of this care is expensive, and neither insurance companies nor the medical establishment wants to pay for it. The U.S. model of medicine is less effective at providing long-term care and giving chronically ill people the medications, equipment, and training in day-to-day self-care they need to stay as healthy as possible.

For a directory of disease management resources, see the website of the Disease Management Association: www.dmaa.org.

The uninsured

According to the U.S. Census Bureau, in 2004, 45.8 million people or 15.7 percent of the U.S. population had no health insurance. That's one out of every six people. Eleven percent (or 8.3 million) of the uninsured were under 18. Seventy percent of the uninsured had at least one full-time worker in their family. Sixty-six percent were families living in poverty. Minorities, who comprise 34 percent of the population, made up 52 percent of the uninsured.

Most people who are uninsured remain so because their employers do not offer it, they do not or cannot work, they cannot afford health insurance, they do not qualify for state-sponsored or low-income insurance (even if they cannot afford any other insurance) or they have a preexisting condition. If you do not get a group premium through an employer, insurers in the individual market may deny coverage or charge higher premiums to people they believe will have high medical costs, such as the chronically ill. This is especially frightening for those of us with hep C, since the treatments for our disease can be very costly, and we may be unable to work due to sickness or debilitating fatigue.

Georgetown University has a great site that offers state-by-state Consumer Guides to Getting and Keeping Health Insurance. These consumer guides are free, and you can read them online or in PDF format. They also have other free guides you can download, such as Understanding Private Health Insurance, Medicare and Medicaid: A Health Care Safety Net for People with Serious Disabilities and Chronic Conditions, and Options for Avoiding and Managing Medical Debt. You can find all of this at: www.healthinsuranceinfo.net/.[1]

Federal health insurance

There are three types of government health insurance: Medicare, Medicaid, and veterans' health benefits. All three will cover medical expenses for hepatitis C, although they may not cover visits to specialists, and the health care you receive may not be as good as what you would receive through a high-end private insurance plan. Call the numbers below for detailed, up-to-date information.

○ If you're 65, you are eligible for **Medicare.** This means you will finally get back the money you paid in Social Security and Medicare taxes. You can sign up for Medicare at a nearby Social Security office.

Medicare has a separate plan for prescription drugs. Medicare is also available to those under 65 who have collected Social Security Disability Insurance (SSD or SSDI) for 24 months. To find out more about Medicare, call 800-MEDICARE, or go to www.medicare.gov/ or www.cms.hhs.gov/

○ Medicaid is a federal-state program providing health care for people with low incomes. **Medicaid** is based on need and covers major medical health conditions and prescriptions. In each state, there is an eligibility scale as to the amount of income you can earn in order to qualify for Medicaid, so in addition to being either age 65 or older or disabled you must demonstrate that your income and assets are low enough to qualify. Call your county social services department to find out if you are eligible. You can also find information at www.cms.hhs.gov/

○ Veterans may also receive medical benefits and disability. Call 800-827-1000 to be connected to the Veterans Benefits Administration Regional Office or go to www.vba.va.gov.

Government disability insurance

Getting disability insurance is a complicated process. It's not unusual to be denied coverage at first. You need to be persistent, and many people recommend getting a lawyer to help you. In most cases, 25 percent of your first disability check goes to pay the lawyer, unless your lawyer waives your fee. For up-to-date information on disability programs, call the Social Security Administration at 800-772-1213. The Administration offers two programs: SSDI and SSI.

○ SSDI (Social Security Disability Insurance) covers workers who have been working for long enough to have made enough contributions to their Social Security accounts.

○ SSI (Supplemental Security Income) provides payments for people who are disabled or 65 and older and have little or no income or financial resources. One of the problems with disability is that, once you qualify, you can't earn over a certain income per year, or they'll take your disability payment away from you.

"It took me a year to get permanent and total disability. In addition to a letter from my doctor, I needed to fill out all of these government forms and so did my friends. I got a lawyer to help me with it. It still took a year, and that's really typical. I was sick and had no income. All of this red tape just for a few hundred dollars a month."

—OLIVIA J.

Choosing an insurance plan

Make sure the plan covers the doctor or doctors you want to see. There are group plans that don't allow you to choose a doctor and send you to a different doctor every time. These plans are a little cheaper, but if you have hep C, it's important for you to be able to establish an ongoing relationship with a doctor who is knowledgeable about hep C and will work hand-in-hand with you to monitor your health. It's also important for you to be able to see specialists, such as hepatologists, gastroenterologists, and transplant physicians. Make sure your plan covers them.

Types of insurance

○ Managed care (HMOs and PPOs) cover your medical expenses only on the condition that you see a doctor who belongs to their network. Some plans allow you to see doctors outside the network, but you have to pay a higher percentage of the fee.

○ PPOs generally allow you to choose any doctor in the network.

○ HMOs require that you choose a primary care physician (PCP) and won't pay for health care provided by other doctors unless your PCP refers you to them.

○ Fee for service. This is the old kind of insurance. It's a lot less common now. With this kind of insurance, you're free to choose your doctor, but the monthly premium may be higher.

Guidelines for Choosing Insurance

○ Be sure to read the entire policy before signing it. If you have any questions, be sure to ask someone. Your insurance agent or the human relations person at your company should be able to help you.

O If you are a freelancer you may want to talk to some of your colleagues who may be in similar work situations. As we mentioned above, there are many unions for freelancers. Small business owners may want to contact their local Small Business Administration office. If you know someone who is a human relations person at a larger company, they may also be able to lend advice.

O Check the restrictions on your policy. Will it cover experimental treatments, such as new kinds of interferon, which are still in clinical trials? If you get sick or injured when you're out of town, does your policy cover visits to doctors and hospitals outside your area? Does it cover emergency room visits?

Be sure to consider the following factors in selecting an insurance plan:

O Monthly premium: Cost per month

O Annual deductible: How much you have to pay out of pocket before the insurance company pays. If you're relatively young and healthy, it may be worth choosing a policy with a large deductible, because you'll pay a much lower premium. The risk is that if you get seriously injured or sick, you'll most likely end up paying a lot more. If you're older or have a higher risk of serious illness, your best bet is to get a policy with a low deductible.

O Coinsurance: Usually your insurance company pays 70 to 80 percent and you pay 20 to 30 percent, but the insurance pays 100 percent after you have paid a certain amount called the "out-of-pocket maximum." You should find out what this out-of-pocket maximum is.

O Policy maximum (cap): the maximum amount the policy will pay during your lifetime. Find out what this is. One million may sound like a huge amount of money, but when you have a chronic condition, your lifetime medical expenses can add up to a lot more than that.

O "Reasonable and customary fee schedule": Many policies retain the right to decide if your doctor or hospital is charging too much money, and they may refuse to pay "unreasonable rates." If your policy contains this clause, you might want to check with a friend or coworker who has the same policy. Ask if his or her insurance has ever refused to pay doctor's bills on the grounds of "unreasonable rates." Under what circumstances?

Ways to get free medical care

FREE DRUG PROGRAMS

Many pharmaceutical companies sponsor "compassionate care" programs for people who can't afford the drugs they need. Usually your doctor has to petition the drug company, fill out paperwork, and reapply every three months. For information, ask your doctor to call the Pharmaceutical Research Manufacturers of America (202-835-4300).

○ The Free Medicine Program (800-921-0072) helps people get prescriptions free of charge.
○ Call the Federal Hill-Burton Free Care Program (800-638-0742) to ask about free programs at hospitals. You can also write to: 5600 Parklawn Bldg., Room 10C-16, Rockville, MD 20857. It is often useful to provide a self-addressed stamped envelope whenever you are requesting information.
○ Call the DEL-Federal Bureau of Primary Health Care (301-594-4100) to ask about free care at their health care centers.
○ Call the Schering-Plough Commitment to Care (800-521-7157) for information on receiving free interferon treatment. If you are having a difficult time getting your insurance company to cover your interferon therapy, these people may go to bat for you.

CLINICAL TRIALS

One way to get free blood tests, physical exams, and pharmaceuticals is to participate in a clinical trial. Most of these trials are sponsored by pharmaceutical companies. The FDA requires that these companies test their drugs before these products can go on the market. The drug companies give you lots of blood tests and other medical exams to see if you meet their criteria for the trial. Many of them have very stringent requirements. They may exclude you based on one of the test results, if your liver enzymes are too high or too low, for instance. Lisa tried to get into a clinical trial in 1996, but she was excluded because she was very slightly anemic. Nonetheless, she got expensive tests for free, including a viral load test and a biopsy.

Be sure to check out the trial before you enroll. Many people have benefited from these trials. They help researchers learn more about hepatitis C. But the primary goal is to test the drug, not to treat the patient. Be sure to find out everything you can about the drug and its side effects. Most drugs being tested to treat hepatitis C include interferon, which has severe side effects. It's always wise to get second and third opinions from doctors not involved in the study and talk to people who have taken the drug before you enroll.

CenterWatch Clinical Trials Listing Service
www.centerwatch.com

Information on clinical trials
www.clinicaltrials.com

RESEARCH STUDIES

Another way to get free health care is to enroll in a research study. These studies are often conducted by top-notch researchers who are receiving government grants to study hepatitis C. Your doctor can recommend you as a participant for a National Institute of Health (NIH) research study. Ask your doctor to call the Warren Grant Magnuson Clinical Center's Patient Referral Services Unit (301-496-2563) or write to:

National Institutes of Health
Bethesda, MD 20892-7511

As in clinical trials, the doctors will give you free medical tests to see if you qualify for the study, and if you do, you can get free pharmaceutical drugs.

Before you enroll in a clinical trial or research study, ask yourself the following questions:

- ○ What are the side effects of the treatment?
- ○ Can you drop out of the study?
- ○ Are you doing it for the free medical tests or for the drug?
- ○ Will you get the drug you want, or is there a chance you'll be part of a "control group," given a placebo? Even if you do get a placebo, some trials will give you the drug they're studying after the trial. You'll get the same amount of the drug, only later. Find out if this is the case.

Financial planning

"My partner and I recently discovered that we both have hep C. We have two small children, and we have no idea how we're going to support them if we both get sick and can't work. How are we even going to support ourselves?"

—DAVID Z.

As we've said before, when you have hep C, it's a good policy to hope for the best but prepare for the worst. Chances are you'll outlive the disease, but it's never wise to assume you'll never have to worry about money.

A few guidelines include:

○ Save your money. Many people who work take a percentage from every paycheck and deposit it in a retirement fund. Your company may already have set one up for you. The IRS takes a small percentage of your income and sets it aside for Social Security. But this money is usually not enough to live on, and you don't want to rely on it. Social Security may not be around when you retire.

○ Figure out your budget. Break your expenses down into categories: food, rent or mortgage payments, car payments, insurance, gasoline, health costs, entertainment, etc. Keep track of all your expenses for a month. This will help you figure out how you can reduce your expenses in some areas and save money.

○ Be sure your money is in a safe place—in the bank, not under your mattress.

○ It's a good idea to keep enough money in your savings account to pay for three months living expenses in case you lose your job or other sources of income. Be sure that this money is easily accessible. If you buy shares of stock or deposit your money in an IRA, it may take a while to access your money if you need it.

Use common sense when planning for your future. Even if you can only save a tiny amount, this is better than nothing.

IN A SENTENCE:

> *Health insurance is necessary when you have a chronic illness. If you have health insurance, find out the details of your plan; if you don't have health insurance, you need to shop around.*

WEEK 3

living

Dealing with Depression and Coping with Illness

THERE'S NO doubt that a positive attitude can make a huge difference in how we feel—and in our actual health. But it's hard to feel positive about having hep C. We were both really upset when we received our diagnoses, but this is different from being chronically depressed. There's nothing unusual about feeling sad when you find out you have a chronic illness. Suddenly you have to live with the knowledge that you may never be perfectly healthy again, and you have to change your life. You may have to stop drinking, for instance, and this may make you feel like an outsider in some situations. At first, it may seem almost impossible to adjust to your new life, and you may feel as if no one understands what you're going through. You may need to find some other people with hep C who do understand. Cara was very lucky to have met Lisa while she was going through her first reactions to her illness. She was extremely sad and felt very isolated. Lisa helped her look at the positive sides of the illness and begin accepting it.

This initial sadness is very common. We all go through a period of mourning, and feeling our sadness and anger is far better than denying that they're there. Grief is the path to accepting our illness. We may have to mourn before we can get on with our lives.

TRY THIS

Write the story of how you found out you have hep C, and how you're dealing with the news. You can use the following questions as guidelines.

- ◯ How did you find out that you have hep C?
- ◯ How did you feel when you first found out?
- ◯ Review the section in Day 1 on the five stages of grief—denial, anger, bargaining, depression, and acceptance. Do you feel as if you've gone through any of these stages? Remember that you won't necessarily go through them in order, and you can experience more than one at once. Which stages are the most familiar? What feelings are the strongest? What experiences trigger those feelings now?
- ◯ What was especially difficult for you to accept and adjust to? What is still difficult to accept?

If you are feeling sad, give yourself time. On the other hand, if you find that you experience drastic changes that last for months, you may be suffering from clinical depression. We strongly encourage you to seek help if you are experiencing a sustained and significant change involving any of the following symptoms. Many people also report these as symptoms of hep C. No matter what, you may still want to get help.

- ◯ Fatigue
- ◯ Loss of interest in activities you usually enjoy
- ◯ Change in sleep patterns
- ◯ Rapid, unexplained weight loss
- ◯ Loss of appetite
- ◯ Weepiness
- ◯ Thoughts about suicide
- ◯ Feelings of worthlessness, helplessness, or loss of hope.

Seeking help for depression

If you are experiencing symptoms of depression, we encourage you to seek out therapy and build a strong support network. Trusted friends and doctors can often recommend a good therapist or support group. Some of us may prefer to find a support group for people with hep C.

While it's important to mourn following your diagnosis, it's also important to realize that hep C is not the end of your life. Having a chronic illness can help you learn to take care of yourself and put things in perspective.

How we cope with illness: Examining our family patterns

"I had been having a really hard time dating. I felt weird because of my hep C. I have always been the caretaker, and I didn't want to put someone in the position where they had to take care of me. But at my hep C support group I met the greatest guy who understood everything I was going through. It's different when we are both worried about taking care of each other."

—SARA B.

"I was raised as a Christian Scientist. My parents don't believe in going to the doctor or in getting medication to treat anything. My grandfather died of diabetes, because he never went to the doctor and never found out. I've worked my entire adult life in getting away from my Christian Science background and getting rid of a lot of baggage. In 1987, when I was in my early 30s, I was in a car accident and rushed to the hospital from the accident scene. When I woke up, I discovered they had given me a blood transfusion to save my life. A few years later I tried to give blood and found out I had gotten hep C from my 1987 transfusion. Even though I don't believe in Christian Science, it's hard for me to go to

the doctor and get regular tests. Since I don't
have symptoms, my family doesn't believe that there is
anything wrong with me."

—GREGORY S.

Being diagnosed with a chronic illness can bring up a lot of issues that you might not have known you have. Many of us have preconceived notions that

○ illness means we're contaminated or dirty
○ we did something wrong and brought our illness upon ourselves
○ it's selfish to ask for what we need
○ we don't have the right to be sick, or to take time to care for ourselves.

Any of these assumptions can seriously interfere with our health.

When you have a chronic condition like hep C, it's crucial to examine your patterns of dealing with illness, as well as your preconceived notions of disease. A good way to get in touch with these patterns is to ask yourself how your family of origin treated you when you were sick? How did they treat themselves?

○ Did people in your family take good care of themselves when they were sick? Did they take good care of you when you were sick as a child?
○ Did they take sick days? What was their general attitude toward sick days? Did they work 10 years without a single day off, or did they spend the day in bed at the first sign of a cold?
○ How did your family respond when you told them you were sick? As a child? As a teenager? As an adult?
○ Were the people in your family able to ask for what they needed, or did they have a hard time asking for help?
○ When and if they asked for help, how were they treated? Did other people try to meet their needs?
○ Did you ever care for someone who was seriously ill? How did you feel about it? Has someone cared for you when you were seriously ill? How did you feel about that?

○ Do you feel as if people in your family complained a lot about illness? Did they tell you (or tell each other) to stop complaining?

○ How did your family deal with serious illness? Did they talk about it? How?

○ How did they deal with death? Did they talk about death? How?

○ Do you recognize any patterns in the way you handle illness as an adult? How do you handle sickness in your partner or spouse? In your friends? Your children?

○ Can you see any behavior patterns that no longer serve you? How can you change these patterns? Who can you enlist to help you in this process?

"When I was a kid, my mother put me to bed at the first sign of a cold. I used to get all of these rewards for being sick, like special treatment and staying home from school. As soon as I found out I had hep C, I started getting extremely fatigued and wanting to use the hep C as an excuse to stay home from work. I'm afraid I'm making up my symptoms. I'm trying to look at this in therapy."

—JASON W.

Asking for what you need

The process of identifying family patterns provides us with important information about how we take care of ourselves, including whether we can ask for help. Whether we're sick or healthy, none of us is entirely self-sufficient. But many of us have lived relatively independent lives as adults. It can be hard for us to ask for help. For some of us—especially those who are very ill—this may be the first time in our lives that we truly have to turn to other people for help, and learn to ask for what we need. But asking for what we need increases our chances of getting it. When Cara was going through her seroconversion illness, she was so sick that she lost her job. She had to turn to her family for some financial support and to her friends to provide company and to help her do things like shop for groceries. The first step in asking for what we need is to recognize when the need arises. We can learn to identify our needs by paying careful attention to our emotions.

The next time you feel anxious or overwhelmed, try asking yourself:

- ○ What situation is triggering these feelings?
- ○ What needs could they be signaling?
- ○ What would make this situation easier on you?
- ○ Whom could you ask for help?

Feelings of anxiety can tip us off to the fact that we're trying to control something that we can't control. It's important to identify those things and let go of them. Unfortunately this is easier said than done.

- ○ Make a list of things you want to control but can't. It's often hard to admit that we can't control all of the circumstances and people in our lives, but our lives become much less frustrating when we aren't constantly trying to do the impossible.
- ○ What are you ready to let go of? How can you make this process easier on yourself?

IN A SENTENCE:

> *It's common to feel sad about having hep C, but if signs of depression persist, seek help.*

learning

Building a
Support System

*"I have hep C, and I'm pretty sure my partner
does because he has elevated liver enzymes. He's
really in denial about it and won't get tested.
It's really bothering me, because we could be
going through this together."*

—JACKIE C.

ONCE WE'VE identified our needs and can ask for help,
it's important to know which people in our lives are most available to help us and under which circumstances.

Make a list of friends and family members who are supportive.

○ Who can you turn to when things get rough?
○ Who encourages you to share your feelings and listens
to them?
○ Who doesn't judge you harshly no matter what you say?
○ Who wishes the best for you?
○ Who is available when you need him or her?
○ Who is really there for you?
○ Whom do you trust?

O Who keeps your confidences?

Now ask yourself:

O Do you have enough supportive people in your life? Make sure you're not just counting on one person. It's impossible for one person to meet all your needs, even if that person loves you and has the best intentions.

After you list the supportive people in your life, look at each name on the list and ask yourself.

O When has this friend helped you in the past?
O Under which circumstances is he or she especially helpful?
O Under which circumstances is it better to go to someone else?

Now make a list of people who are not very supportive.

O Who doesn't listen well?
O Who says that you complain too much?
O Who says that your feelings aren't real?

Some of these may be people you love, and people who love you. Nonetheless, these are not the best people to go to when you need support. Some names will appear on both lists, since some people are supportive in some circumstances and not in others.

Finding other people with hep C: online and in person

You may have the most supportive family and friends in the world, but unless they've been diagnosed with hep C themselves, they may have a hard time understanding what you're going through. The people who will understand what you're going through are other people who have been diagnosed with hep C.

The two fastest ways to meet other people with hep C are on the Internet and at support groups. At first you may feel weird about turning to strangers for help. But these people have a lot to offer, including empathy, information, and a variety of viewpoints on the latest treatments and ways of dealing with the day-to-day hardships of living with hep C. No matter how severe your symptoms are, you will find people who can relate. Some people will be inspiring and others will be discouraging, but either way, you will learn that it's possible to live with hep C. Meeting other people with hep C will help you accept your diagnosis and come to terms with the fact that you have hep C.

The World Wide Web

If you're researching a new treatment or study, you'll want to look on the World Wide Web. The Web is easily accessible from your home.

There are hundreds of Web sites devoted solely to hepatitis C. Google, Ask Jeeves, Yahoo!, and Alta Vista are some popular search engines. You can use these to look up information on the Internet. Many Web sites are updated daily. As we discuss in Month 7, "Keeping Up to Date and Doing Research," this is an excellent source for breaking news.

Places to start:

○ American Liver Foundation: www.liverfoundaton.org
○ Hep-C-Alert: www.hep-c-alert.org/
○ American Association for the Study of Liver Diseases: www.aasld.org
○ Ask Doc Misha: www.docmisha.com
○ CDC Emerging Diseases Page: www.cdc.gov/ncidod/EID/index.htm
○ Web site of former Surgeon General Dr. C. Everett Koop: Epidemic.org
○ HCV Advocate: www.hcvadvocate.org
○ Hep C Advocate Network: www.hepcan.org
○ Hepatitis C Society of Canada: www.web.idirect.com/~hepc
○ Hepatitis Webring—links to hepatitis sites: f.webring.com/hub?ring=hepring
○ Hepatitis-central.com
○ www.HepCPrimer.com
○ Hepatitis Directory of Online Resources: www.objectivemedcine.com/dbsearch.htm

○ HepNet—The Hepatitis Information Network—a source for both doctors and patients about viral hepatitis: www.hepnet.com

○ Hepatology Watch: www.hepwatch.com

Newsgroups

You can sign up for a hepatitis C newsgroup. One good newsgroup is USENET sci.med.diseases.hepatitis. When you sign up for a newsgroup, this gives you access to a Web page that is like a bulletin board. The board contains the titles of messages that people have posted. You click on a title to read the message. If you reply to the message, your reply will be posted on the bulletin board, where the other members of the newsgroup can see the title and click on it to read your reply. One site that has a bulletin board is www.hepatitis-central.com. There is also a bulletin board for veterans with hep C at hcvets.com. To find more newsgroups, do a search on a major search engine, such as Google or Yahoo!, for "hepatitis C newgroups."

E-mail lists: Inbox delivery

An e-mail list is a lot like a newsgroup, except that, when you subscribe to an e-mail list, all the messages that the other members write are sent directly to your inbox. Likewise, if you reply to a message, your reply is sent to everyone on the list. E-mail lists generally have rules of what you can and cannot post, and some lists have moderators who screen every message before posting it and weed out a lot of junk mail and other messages that aren't appropriate for the list. Some e-lists have archives, which allow you to search for topics that were posted before you subscribed.

E-lists are a valuable source of information and support. You can ask questions about hep C and get immediate response from other members—often from a wide range of viewpoints. If you don't want to ask questions yourself, you can still benefit from other people's posts. Either way, you will find that other people with hep C have many of the same questions you do, and that there are many ways of dealing with the issues you face. E-lists can also give you a sense of community and remind you that you're not alone.

Hepatitis C Mail List – Hepatitis C News
To subscribe, send an email message to HepC-subscribe@egroups.com

Hepatitis C Advocacy Mail List
To subscribe, go to www.hepcadvocacy.org/emailList.html

Help4HCV List
help4hcv@yahoo.com
www.myspace.com/help4hcv

Chat rooms: Instant communication

In Internet chat rooms, your message is posted as you type, so that everyone in the chat room can read it. This means it's possible to ask a question and get almost instantaneous feedback. But sometimes you have to sit in front of the computer for a long time before anyone responds, and you miss the messages that are posted when you're not in front of your computer screen. The fact that chat rooms are in "real time" can be frustrating when you're looking for information or support.

Some Hep C Chat Rooms:

Janis & Friends Hepatitis C Support Site
www.janis7hepc.com/our_chat_room_and_message_boards.htm

Hep C Palace
www.heppalace.net/

Priority Health Corporation
www.hepatitisneighborhood.com

Support groups: Finding people in the flesh

If you prefer meeting people in person—or if you'd rather talk than type—the best way to meet other people with hep C is to go to a support group at a local hospital or community center. These groups usually meet about once a month and sponsor speakers, such as medical professionals, to talk on some aspect of hepatitis C. These groups offer face-to-face contact and socializing, but since many of them only meet once a month this might not be the best way to get immediate feedback on an urgent question you have.

"When I first got diagnosed with hep C, I didn't know anybody else who had it. I found a support group through my local hospital, and I really hit it off with some of the people

there. It's amazing how much we have in common. We're all from very different walks of life yet hep C brings us together. Some people have really severe symptoms, but other people have the same mild symptoms I do. We talk about how we deal with depression and fatigue. It helps me to know other people are going through the same thing."

—MATT O.

"I've had hep C for a while, but I've never really gone out and talked to people with hep C. I didn't feel like I needed to. When I thought about doing interferon, my doctor suggested that I go talk to people who had been on it. I'm really shy and hate meeting new people, so I found people online first. Then I actually found a support group where I could go and meet the people face-to-face. I met people who were experiencing a whole range of side effects. Some couldn't get out of bed, and some were working full-time just fine. I decided to go on interferon anyway because I'm at Stage 3 fibrosis. One of the best things about the support group was all of the great suggestions I got for how to deal with the side effects. Acupuncture really helps."

—JOYCE A.

Below are some Web sites and phone numbers to help you find local support groups:

Hepatitis-central.com
www.hepatitis-central.com/hcv/support/main.html (Lists worldwide support groups as well.)

HepCPrimer.com
www.hepcprimer.com/patient/support.html

Objective Medicine
www.objectivemedicine.com

Priority Healthcare Corporation
www.hepatitisneighborhood.com

Hepatitis A, B, and C Prevention Programs
Lists many different support groups
www.hepprograms.org/support/hepc.asp

IN A SENTENCE:

> *Meeting other people with hep C can help you understand what you are going through.*

Thinking about Your Treatment Options

"I am thinking about going into treatment. I'm young, and this is a huge decision. Do I go on and possibly give up a year of my life now in the hopes that there is a chance I might clear the virus? Or do I continue living the way I am with the thought that I might never get sick? I'm hesitant to start anything until I make my decision."

—CARA BRUCE

NOW, BY your fourth week of living with hep C, you've dealt with the shock and started making changes. You may be ready to consider your treatment options. Considering how fast research and treatments for hep C are changing, it's important to keep abreast of new treatments. There are a number of ways to do this: You can begin by researching on the Web and getting on e-lists devoted to hep C. Search the hep C sites, as well as major newspapers and periodicals. Many organizations like the American Liver Foundation (ALF) have compiled current articles. However, just because an article is in the newspaper doesn't mean it's correct. Chat rooms and support groups are also good forums for talking to people who have been through treatment, but remember that the people in chat rooms are rarely professionals. Whatever you find, it's a good idea to double-check with at least a few sources and ask your doctor before you try any new treatment. This is one of the reasons why it's important to find a doctor who's available to discuss these things with you. Some conventional western doctors may scoff at acupuncture and other alternative treatments. If you're interested in researching or pursuing these treatments, find specialists in this area or western doctors who know about or practice the treatments you're interested in.

You may find some conflicting information, especially on the Web, but don't let this scare you. We provide guidelines for finding and evaluating information in Month 7, "Keeping Up to Date and Doing Research," and in the resource section we've included a list of reliable Web sites to help you. A lot of these Web sites also have hotlines you can call to ask more in-depth questions.

Below is a list of hepatitis organizations that you can call to ask about treatment options and referrals:

American Liver Foundation (ALF)
75 Maiden Lane
Suite 603
New York, NY 10038
800-GO-LIVER (465-4837)
800-4HEP-USA (443-7872)
www.liverfoundation.org

HCV Advocate
P.O. Box 427037
San Francisco, CA 94142-7037
www.hcvadvocate.org
alanfranciscus@hcvadvocate.org

Hep-C Alert
660 NE 125 Street
North Miami, FL 33161
954-920-5277
Toll-Free: 877-HELP-4-HEP
877-435-7443
Fax: 305-893-7998
www.hep-c-alert.org

Hepatitis Foundation International
504 Blick Drive
Silver Spring, MD 20904-2901
800-891-0707
www.hepfi.org
hfi@comcast.net

The Hep C Connection
Hep C Hotline: 800-522-HEPC
www.hepc-connection.org

These drug companies can provide information on various treatments:

Valeant Pharmaceuticals
www.infergen.com
877-361-2719
Infergen Aspire: 24/7 Nursing Support and Reimbursement Program
888-MOVE-FWD

"Be in Charge" Program
Schering Oncology Biotech
888-437-2608
www.beincharge.com

Schering-Plough's Commitment to Care Program
Sliding Scale Program
800-521-7157

Federal Hill-Burton Free Care Program
5600 Parklawn Bldg. Room 10C-16
Rockville, MD 20857
Free Care Program (800-638-0742)
Bureau of Primary Health Care (301-594-4100)

PegIntron (Schering Plough's pegylated interferon)
www.PegIntron.com
888-437-2608

Ribavirin
www.nlm.nih.gov/medlineplus/druginfo/uspdi/202509.html
www.hepatitis-central.com/hcv/ribavirin/toc.html

Hoffman-LaRoche
www.roche.com/home/diseases/dis_hep.htm
www.pegasys.com
PegAssist is the Pegasys information program
877-PEG-ASYS (734-2797)
Roche Biocare's financial assistance line
800-443-6676

Below are sites that can offer medical advice and help you do research:

CenterWatch Clinical Trials Listing Service
www.centerwatch.com

Information on clinical trials
www.clinicaltrials.com

Medline—US National Library of Medicine (NLM)
World's largest database of medical literature.
www.nlm.NIH.gov/medlineplus

Medscape
www.medscape.com

How to spot scams

> *"I saw a flyer posted on a telephone pole by my house boasting: 'Miracle Cure for Hep C: Selenium.' I went out and bought a bottle of selenium. Then I looked up the 'miracle cure' Web site, and it was this crazy site with all of these political rants that made no sense. Like selenium was going to cause world peace. I got worried because I thought my selenium might not be good for anything at all. But then I did more searches on the Web and found out that selenium was good for hep C, it just wasn't a miracle cure."*
>
> —MARCY P.

As a person who's just acquired a chronic illness, it's important to realize that you may be a target for con artists who prey on people who are desperate for an answer. It's OK to feel out of control. We all want a cure for hepatitis C, but it's important to be able to distinguish between treatments that can help, and scams, which just eat up your money.

While there's no one guaranteed way to spot a scam, there are some things to watch out for:

O Does the treatment make blanket statements or sweeping generalizations?

O Does it claim to be 100 percent effective for everyone? No treatment works for everyone all the time.

○ In the same vein, does the treatment claim to cure all ills? Does it claim that one factor causes everything from cancer to mental illness? Does it claim that you'll live to be 150 years old?

○ Most important, do they ask you to send money?

Check out www.quackwatch.com for the latest scams.

IN A SENTENCE:

> *It's important to consider your treatment options and keep abreast of new research.*

learning

Introduction to Conventional Western Treatments

"It's hard to eat on interferon. But if I eat and drink lots of water, the side effects seem easier to handle. It's also hard to exercise, but I do as much as I can because it makes me feel better. There are some hard things about it, but overall, it's not as bad as I thought it would be."

—IVAN T.

"I am on combination therapy. It's not great, but it's not as bad as I expected. My major worry is that I will not be a sustained responder, and I might not be. Sometimes I wonder why I'm putting myself through this when it could do me absolutely no good."

—ROGER W.

CONVENTIONAL TREATMENTS for hep C are becoming more effective all the time. But so far, there is no treatment that works for the majority of people with hepatitis C. If you decide to pursue treatment, you have to find what works best for you, although you should be sure to check with your doctor before trying anything. Other people with hep C are also an invaluable source of information. They can offer suggestions on which treatments work for them and how they dealt with various symptoms. If you are considering treatment, you may want to join a support group for people with hep C. This is even more important if you're considering conventional drug therapy, which often has severe side effects. Other patients may be able to suggest ways of dealing with these side effects, as well as alternative treatment options you may not have considered.

Conventional western medicine uses two main forms of treatment for hep C:

○ Drug therapy. In the following section we discuss how pharmaceuticals are tested for safety and efficacy and which medications have been approved for the treatment of hepatitis C.
○ Surgery. Liver transplantation is a last-resort procedure, which can prolong the lives of patients who would otherwise die of liver failure. We discuss liver transplants in the Learning section of Month 9.

As of right now, drug therapy includes both pegylated interferon alone (monotherapy) and pegylated interferon in combination with **ribavirin**. So far, these interferon-based therapies are the only treatments that have been shown to eliminate the virus in clinical trials.

Traditionally the drug interferon was injected three times a week, but in 2001, the FDA approved a time-release interferon called **pegylated interferon**, which only has to be injected once a week. Two pharmaceutical companies make pegylated interferon: Schering-Plough's PEG-Intron comes in a prefilled syringe, and Roche's Pegasys comes in a prefilled pen. The dose depends on the patient's weight. Combination therapy lasts for 24 to 72 weeks, with an average of 48 depending on response and genotype. The two main types of ribavirin used in combination therapy are Roche's Copegus and Schering-Plough's Rebetol. Patients take four to six 200 mg tablets of ribavirin per day. In 2005, Three Rivers Pharmaceuticals received FDA approval for Ribasphere. These tablets come in 200 mg, 400 mg, and 600 mg tablets, so patients can take fewer tablets each day.

What is interferon?

Our body produces interferons naturally. When a virus invades one of our cells, the white blood cells and other immune cells produce proteins called interferons, which "interfere" with the production of new virus particles. Interferons have several functions. While they fight viruses, they also play a role in combating cancers and regulating the immune system (a function known a immunomodulatory activity). They may also reverse fibrosis, or scarring of the liver due to HCV or other viruses.

When the body does not produce enough natural interferon to fight an infection such as hep C, the patient may benefit from synthetically produced interferon supplements, which are usually injected under the skin or into the muscle.[1]

In the late 1970s, scientists started using interferon produced by the body to make a drug for treating diseases. At first they derived it from blood. Since then, pharmaceutical companies have manufactured derivatives of interferon, and some of these drugs are currently used to treat hepatitis C.

In 1988, the FDA approved interferon for treating non-A non-B hepatitis. It was approved for hep C in 1991. In 2001, as mentioned above, the FDA approved a time-release interferon called pegylated interferon, which only has to be injected once a week. "Pegylation" is the process of adding a molecule of polyethylene glycol to interferon. The polyethylene glycol acts like a suit of armor: which releases the interferon slowly, and patients only have to inject the drug once a week, rather than three times a week.

What is ribavirin?

Ribavirin is a synthetic antiviral medication. It is not known exactly how ribavirin fights viruses, or why it is only effective against hep C when taken in a "cocktail" with alpha interferon. When taken alone, ribavirin has no effect on HCV RNA, but in combination therapy, ribavirin potentiates interferon's antiviral and immune-boosting activity—producing much higher sustained-response rates than interferon alone. In the current standard treatment for hep C, patients take ribavirin orally at a dose of 800 to 1200 mg per day. Because ribavirin often causes anemia, patients with heart conditions or histories of anemia are generally not considered for treatment. Ribavirin is also excreted through the kidneys, so it should not be used by people with renal problems.

The Recommended Treatment

Studies have shown that the combination of **pegylated interferon** and **ribavirin** is the most effective FDA-approved treatment for hepatitis C. The standard therapy for genotype 1a or 1b is a combination of pegylated interferon and ribavirin for 48 weeks, although therapy may last anywhere from 24 to 72 weeks. People with types 2 and 3, who are more likely to have sustained response to treatment, take combination therapy for an average of 24 weeks. Patients get tested regularly to see if they're responding. Since the side effects of these medications can be severe, most doctors discontinue treatment if the patient doesn't respond or stops responding.

Many promising new drugs such as protease inhibitors are currently in clinical trials. See Month 3, Trends in Research and Treatment, for more information.

Who gets recommended for treatment

Patients are recommended for treatment on a very individual basis. Some doctors tend to recommend treatment much more frequently than others. Indications for treatment include:

○ Positive result on PCR test—indicating viral activity
○ Recent infection. Early treatment may prevent hep C from becoming chronic—provided that the patient starts interferon-based therapy within the first several months of infection.
○ Genotype 2 or 3—the genotypes most likely to respond to treatment
○ Patient's motivation. Interferon can have severe side effects, and many people have a hard time tolerating therapy. A patient with lots of motivation is more likely to tolerate treatment, and patients who take their medication at least 80 percent of the time have a better chance of responding to treatment.

O Advanced liver disease–stage 2 fibrosis or greater

O Severe symptoms

O Emotional and mental stability. People with a history of mental illness can be treated. They just need to be watched more carefully. Many people take antidepressants or other psychiatric medications while they are on interferon.

O Coinfection. Doctors are now urging patients coinfected with HIV and HCV to try combination therapy to eliminate HCV or improve the health of their livers. See Month 11 for more information about treatment for coinfected people.

Methadone and bupenorphine don't affect the success rate of therapy, so patients on these drugs don't need to stop taking them before they receive treatment. The CDC recommends that no one be denied treatment.

Genotype is one of the most important indications for treatment, because patients with genotypes 2 and 3 have a much higher rate of responding to therapy. Even with the most effective drug combo (pegylated interferon and ribavirin), patients with genotype 1 have at most a 52 percent chance of **sustained viral response (SVR)**. A sustained viral response means that the patient has an undetectable viral load in the blood 6 months following the end of treatment. African-Americans are less likely to respond to treatment than other ethnic groups. More studies are needed to determine why this is the case and what can be done about it.

The decision to treat must be made on an individual basis. As we mentioned above, the patient's motivation makes a huge difference. A patient who wants to be treated is far more likely to take the medication.

As we have discussed, only 10 to 20 percent of hep C patients develop cirrhosis. It usually takes 20 to 30 years for this condition to become so severe that it compromises liver function. Many doctors recommend treatment for the patients with the greatest risk of developing cirrhosis. These patients generally have persistently high ALT levels and a liver biopsy that indicates changes under the microscope: the degree of fibrosis (scarring) is stage 2 or greater on a scale of 0 to 4. Since interferon can have severe side effects, many patients with stage 0 or 1 fibrosis choose not to pursue treatment immediately but to lead a healthy lifestyle and wait for new drugs to gain approval. Lisa has decided to do this. She has considered pursuing treatment, but she has genotype 1a, which decreases her chances of sustained response. At the moment she is waiting for more effective medications with less severe side effects. Nonetheless, she keeps up with the latest advances in treatment and discusses the potential risks and benefits with her doctors. For many of us, pursuing treatment is a big decision. It's not something you decide in one day. It's good to learn as much as you can about the medications and weigh your options.

Who can't take interferon

There are a number of health conditions that may prevent you from taking interferon. We list a few below, but it's up to your doctor to evaluate whether or not you can take this drug.

- O **Decompensated cirrhosis**, meaning cirrhosis with symptoms, in contrast to "compensated" or asymptomatic cirrhosis
- O Pregnancy
- O Psychiatric illness. As mentioned above, people with a history of mental illness can be treated; they just need to be watched more carefully. Many people on interferon take antidepressants or other psychiatric medications.
- O Anemia
- O Heart disease
- O Kidney disease
- O Autoimmune disorders
- O Thyroid disorders
- O Thrombocytopenia—meaning a low level of blood platelets, which are needed for clotting.
- O Post-transplant patients.

"I really want to go on the newest pegylated interferon treatment. I have had many drug and alcohol problems in the past, and I'm afraid they will get in my way of being in a clinical trial."

—WILSON S.

Side effects of interferon

A side effect is simply an undesirable effect of a drug or therapy. All medications have some possible side effects. The side effects of interferon are similar to the symptoms of hep C. They are usually most severe at the beginning of treatment, and they abate after you stop taking the drug. Healthy patients are less likely to experience severe side effects. This is a good argument for choosing treatment in the early stages of liver disease, especially if you are genotype 2 or 3 and have a good chance of sustained response. Patients with advanced liver disease or cirrhosis tend to have more debilitating side effects, but they may be able to tolerate the drug better if they start with a lower dose of interferon and build up. If you're thinking of taking interferon, it is important to have a sympathetic doctor who will work with you to reduce side effects so you can get the most out of your treatment. Many patients get acupuncture or other forms of alternative treatment to alleviate the side effects. We suggest a number of other ways to manage side effects below.

Managing the side effects of interferon

FLULIKE SYMPTOMS

Interferon's most common side effects are flulike symptoms, such as fatigue, fever, chills, aching joints, headaches, and weakness. These symptoms tend to be most severe during the first month of treatment, so if you're struggling with these side effects, it is worthwhile to stick it out for more than a month to see if they diminish. The following tips may help relieve flulike symptoms:

○ Drink a gallon of water each day. Staying hydrated is the best thing you can do to relieve flulike symptoms.
○ Take one or two tablets of acetaminophen (Tylenol) half an hour before the interferon shot and four to six hours later. Tylenol has garnered a lot of press for causing liver damage, but it is usually only dangerous when one takes more than 15 grams at once (or at least 7 to 10). Taking four grams (or eight pills) a day according to directions on the label is easier on the liver than nonsteroidal anti-inflammatories (NSAIDs) such as aspirin and ibuprofen, which should be avoided.

○ Some patients find it helpful to inject the interferon 15 to 30 minutes before bedtime. But if the drug disturbs your sleep, you may want to take it in the morning. Thirty to 40 percent of patients on interferon report insomnia, which can aggravate other side effects such as fatigue and depression.

○ Take a warm bath for chills, or use cooling packs for low-grade fever.

○ If hot weather exacerbates flulike symptoms, use air-conditioning.

○ Exercise and massage can help alleviate aches and pains.

FATIGUE

Many people with hepatitis report fatigue, and this symptom does not correspond to the severity of liver disease or damage. Even without hep C or interferon, roughly one in four percent of Americans suffer from fatigue. When you add both hep C and interferon treatments, the numbers increase to 50 percent. Diet and exercise can go a long way toward managing fatigue.

○ Again, drink lots of water.

○ Eat five or six small meals a day, since people tend to become tired after large, heavy meals.

○ Avoid sugar, which will give you a brief rush, then make you more tired.

○ Take naps. Even a 15- or 20-minute nap once or twice a day can help.

○ Exercise. Even if you're exhausted, do 10 minutes a day and build up to more.

○ Get as much sleep as you need. Most people require seven or eight hours.

○ Wake up at the same time every day, regardless of how long you sleep.

○ Bupropion (Wellbutrin), methylphenidate (Ritalin), and modafinil (Provigil) have been used to reduce fatigue in people with HIV and chronic fatigue syndrome. A small study indicated that Ritalin significantly boosted the energy of hep C patients on interferon.

○ Avoid alcohol, a sedative.

○ Quit smoking.

If you experienced fatigue before your interferon treatments, it is worth considering other factors. Treating fatigue is challenging, because there is a wide variety of possible causes. Some contributing factors include:

○ Lack of sleep
○ Depression
○ Stress
○ Lack of exercise
○ Overwork
○ Being overweight
○ Excessive alcohol consumption
○ Excessive caffeine consumption
○ Anemia
○ Poor nutrition (lack of protein or iron, for instance)
○ Electrolyte imbalances (low sodium, for instance)
○ Thyroid disease
○ Other diseases, such as congestive heart failure.

Psychological effects

More than half of the people on interferon report depression or related side effects such as irritability, emotional instability, fatigue, confusion, insomnia, difficulty concentrating, decreased appetite, and weight loss. Between 35 and 57 percent of people with hep C experience these symptoms prior to interferon treatment as a result of a preexisting condition or hep C. Nonetheless, even people who have never been depressed tend to experience some depression on interferon, and these psychological side effects can disrupt a patient's relationships with friends, family, coworkers, and doctors. For this reason, Dr. Melissa Palmer recommends that most patients—even those with no history of psychiatric problems—start taking an antidepressant or antianxiety drug one month prior to beginning treatment. The safest are SSRIs such as Celexa, Lexapro, Prozac, Paxil, or Zoloft and should be started one month before starting interferon therapy. Lexapro takes effect most quickly. Wellbutrin has fewer sexual side effects and can also help patients quit smoking.

INSOMNIA

Many people with liver disease suffer from sleep disorders, and interferon can contribute to them. Thirty to 40 percent of patients on interferon report insomnia. It is important to address this side effect immediately, since it can aggravate other common effects of interferon, such as fatigue, depression, anxiety, and trouble concentrating. Like fatigue, insomnia can be hard to treat due to the wide variety of possible factors. See Day 7 Living: "Getting Exercise and Overcoming Insomnia" for tips on improving your sleep.

SEXUAL SIDE EFFECTS

With flulike symptoms, depression, and fatigue as possible side effects, it's no surprise that some people on interferon find that they are less interested in sex. Some women taking interferon suffer from vaginal dryness, which can cause itching and discomfort, as well as yeast infections and vaginitis (inflammation of the vagina). To relieve vaginal dryness during intercourse, use a water-soluble lubricant. Oil- and petroleum-based lubricants, such as Vaseline, can irritate the vagina, increase the risk of infections, and cause condoms and other latex products to break. Kegel exercises (contracting the same muscles you use to stop the flow of urine) stimulate vaginal lubrication by increasing blood flow to the vagina. These exercises also strengthen the pelvic muscles.

Some men on interferon also experience sexual side effects, such as decreased libido and difficulty having or maintaining erections. The effects of Viagra on people with liver disease and liver transplants has not been sufficiently studied. Since this drug causes abnormal liver function tests in 2 percent of men, it may be worth investigating other treatments for erectile dysfunction. Hep C patients should only take Viagra under a doctor's supervision—which does not mean that the doctor needs to be present when you use it, of course. Many doctors recommend a dose of 25 mg, instead of the usual 50 mg, for patients with liver disease.

Interferon can also cause hair loss, mouth ulcers, and dry skin. These side effects can make patients feel less attractive and consequently less interested in sex. Mucositis, which we discuss below, can cause ulcerations of the mouth, throat, and anus, which can make kissing and sex painful and potentially risky for HCV-free partners. We offer suggestions for managing these side effects below.

MUCOSITIS

The lining, or mucosa, of the gastrointestinal tract, including the mouth, throat, stomach, intestines, and anus, is one of the most sensitive regions of the body. The mucosal cells divide rapidly and have a short lifespan. When a medication, such as interferon, kills these cells, they can take seveb to fourteen days to regenerate. In the meantime, the patient may experience mucositis, an inflammation of the mucosa, and the accompanying symptoms of redness, excessive dryness, raw sores, and a burning sensation that feels like sunburn, except it's internal. This condition, which can occur anywhere from the mouth to anus, can lead to complications such as severe pain, decreased appetite and consequently poor nutrition and weight loss, as well as hemorrhaging and infections, which require prompt antibiotic treatment. The following may help prevent or alleviate mucositis:

○ Practice good oral hygiene. Brush your teeth 3 or 4 times a day, and floss twice a day.
○ Drink fluids consistently and chew sugarless gum to increase the flow of saliva. (Interferon tends to decrease the production of saliva, which kills the bacteria that cause tooth decay.)
○ Apply lip balm to the lips, especially before bedtime. Topical corticosteroids, such as fluocinomide, may also help.
○ Rinse your mouth with baking soda. Avoid commercial mouthwashes that contain alcohol.
○ Anesthetics, such as Xylocaine, and over-the-counter topical solutions, such as Orabase B, can numb painful mouth ulcers.
○ Take care of any dental or periodontal work three to six months before starting interferon or one to three months after finishing the regimen.
○ Quit smoking. It worsens mucositis.

INJECTION-SITE REACTIONS

After an interferon injection, most people experience redness, swelling, itching and soreness at the injection site. This inflammation is more common with pegylated interferon, which is injected once a week, than with the older interferons that require three injections per week. The reaction usually occurs within two days of the injection. The red, swollen area may be an inch in diameter, but if the pain and inflammation become more severe, it's a sign that the injection site may be infected, and the patient should be treated with antibiotics immediately.

○ Before injecting interferon, always clean the injection site with alcohol, Betadine, or another antiseptic. Make sure the alcohol is completely dry before injecting.
○ Make sure the interferon is at room temperature before injecting.
○ Rotate the injection site. For instance, if you're taking pegylated interferon once a week, you can alternate among two sites on your stomach and the right and left thigh. This gives each injection site four weeks to heal.
○ Icing the injection site beforehand may decrease inflammation.
○ Shield the injection site from direct sunlight, which can increase inflammation. Stay out of tanning salons.
○ Hydrocortisone cream and other over-the-counter topical steroids will also reduce inflammation.
○ If the injections are particularly painful, you can request a thinner needle, such as 28- or 29-gauge needle, or mix the interferon with a local anesthetic such as lidocaine.

HAIR LOSS

Interferon is not like chemotherapy. It won't make all your hair fall out, but some patients report minimal thinning. Hair loss seems most frequent in Asians and black-haired Caucasians. It usually occurs three or four months into the treatment. It is always temporary. The hair grows back three to six months after the end of therapy.

To prevent hair loss:

○ Start Nioxin hair-loss treatment a month before starting interferon. You don't need a prescription, and you can purchase it at www.nioxin.com. You can also apply Rogaine topical medication to the scalp.
○ Use a wide-toothed comb.
○ Take the B vitamin biotin daily.

○ Avoid dying, bleaching, permanents, hair-straighteners, curling irons, cornrows, tight ponytails, and braids.

○ Most medical insurances will cover the cost of a wig or hairpiece in a hair emergency.

BONE MARROW SUPPRESSION

The bone marrow produces red blood cells, white blood cells, and platelets. Both hep C and interferon can prevent the bone marrow from producing a sufficient number of these blood cells—leading to low red blood cell count (anemia), low white blood cell count (neutropenia), and low platelet count (thrombocytopenia). These side effects occur most frequently in patients with cirrhosis and in those receiving pegylated interferon. Anemia is more common in people on combination therapy, because it is also a side effect of ribavirin. Thrombocytopenia is less common on combination therapy, because ribavirin causes the reverse condition, elevated platelet counts or thrombocytosis.

Low blood cell counts can be reversed by lowering the dose of interferon, but this can make the treatment less effective. Some medications and supplements may help, but it is crucial that patients with low blood cell counts work with their doctor to maintain the optimal dose of interferon while keeping blood cell counts up.

HYPOTHYROIDISM AND HYPERTHYROIDISM

Roughly 8 percent of people on interferon experience thyroid abnormalities. Symptoms such as weakness, fatigue, weight gain, hair loss, dry skin, memory loss, and psychosis may indicate a slow-functioning thyroid (hypothyroidism). Nervousness, weight loss, heart palpitations, bulging eyes, shortness of breath, poor concentration, and emotional instability may be signs of a fast-functioning thyroid (hyperthyroidism). Both conditions are easy to treat and usually abate when the patient stops taking interferon.[2]

Side effects of ribavirin

Ribavirin has some of the same side effects as interferon, though milder. The number of medications you're taking increases the chance that you'll experience adverse effects, so patients on combination therapy are more likely to have issues with their medications (and discontinue treatment) than those on interferon alone. Also, if you are having side effects, you might want to try some of the nonpharmacological suggestions before you take more medications to offset the effects of your medications.

Managing the side effects of ribivirin

ANEMIA

Ribavirin-induced anemia—a drop in the level of hemoglobin, the iron-rich protein in red blood cells—occurs in 50 to 60 percent of patients on combination therapy and is especially dangerous for people with heart conditions. Men over 40 and women over 50 should have an electrocardiogram (EKG) before starting treatment. The symptoms of anemia, including fatigue, headaches, shortness of breath, and heart palpitations, usually appear during the first few weeks of treatment and cause many patients to stop taking ribavirin.

This condition goes away when people discontinue or decrease their ribavirin dose, but even small reductions in ribavirin can lower one's chance of sustained response by 50 percent. Dr. Melissa Palmer puts patients on supplements—vitamins C (1000 mg) and E (400 to 800 mg)—before they start combination therapy. These vitamins can reduce both the risk and the degree of ribavirin-induced anemia. Studies have shown that Procrit (epoetin alfa), administered subcutaneously at a dose of 40,000 units once a week, raises hemoglobin levels by two to three g/dl, which can improve people's quality of life and help them stay in treatment. Procrit itself can cause fatigue, headaches, fever, high blood pressure, or seizures, but these side effects are infrequent—occurring in only 10 percent of patients.

NAUSEA

Twenty-four to 43 percent of people on combination therapy experience nausea, primarily due to ribavirin. To reduce nausea:

○ Take ribavirin with food.
○ Eat many small meals rather than several large meals.
○ Eat easily digestible foods: crackers, dry toast, broth, Jell-O.
○ Eat a small amount of ginger or drink ginger ale.

○ Don't eat very cold and very hot foods together.
○ Avoid strenuous activity after eating.
○ Rest after meals, but don't lie down.

If none of this works, you can ask your doctor for a prescription for an antinausea medication.

SHORTNESS OF BREATH

Roughly 25 percent of patients on ribavirin report breathlessness or a mild cough. A humidifier or air purifier can help, as can cough suppressants. Since shortness of breath is a symptom of anemia, your doctor will want to order a blood test for hemoglobin level. If this isn't the problem, you may need to have a chest X-ray to eliminate other causes.

SKIN PROBLEMS

Ten to 30 percent of people on ribavirin experience itching, dry skin, or rashes.

For relief from itching:

○ Drink one gallon of water a day.
○ Avoid hot baths and showers.
○ Wear loose-fitting cotton clothes.
○ Use anti-itching soaps and oatmeal-based lotions such as Aveeno, Cetaphil, and L'Occitane.
○ Avoid perfumed soaps and lotions.

If these suggestions don't work, you can also apply Benadryl lotion or hydrocortisone cream to rashes or itchy skin, or take antihistamines such as Benadryl or Claritin.

To prevent sunburns, avoid direct sunlight and use a sunscreen of SPF 30 on exposed skin before going outside during the day.

BIRTH DEFECTS

Ribavirin can cause birth defects, so anyone who is pregnant or wants to get pregnant cannot take it. Doctors generally recommend that patients use two forms of birth control while on ribavirin and for six months following the end of treatment.[3]

How medications get on the market

The drugs that we've just discussed have many side effects and are less effective than we'd like them to be. The treatments for hep C are getting more effective and more tolerable all the time, but it takes a while for new medications to come out on the market. Before a pharmaceutical drug can go on the market, it has to pass clinical trials and be approved by the U.S. Food and Drug Administration (FDA). The FDA monitors the safety and efficacy of a wide variety of food ingredients, pharmaceutical drugs and medical devices. There are advantages and disadvantages to this system.

The advantage is that a drug can only go on the market once it has passed clinical trials, and there is evidence that the drug is safe and effective. Lisa tried to get into a clinical trial in 1996. The trial was for interferon in combination with ribavirin. Most clinical trials are **randomized double-blind placebo-controlled (RDBPC)** studies. This kind of study is considered most scientifically rigorous for establishing the safety and effectiveness of a new kind of treatment. In an RDBPC study, participants are randomly divided into two groups. Some of the participants receive the drug that is being studied, and others (the "control group") take a placebo, a pill that doesn't contain the medication. The participants don't know whether they're getting the drug or not. The study is called "double blind" because their doctors don't know either. The purpose of the control group is to tell whether the medication is having an effect: It's possible that the people would get better anyway, without the medication, or that they would get better because they believed that the drug would cure them.

After the trial, the researchers usually write an article on the results and submit it to a medical journal. Before the journal publishes the paper, it may ask a group of "peers" (other researchers) to evaluate the research and decide whether it's fit for publication. One article or one study usually isn't enough to prove the effectiveness of a drug, but as more trials yield similar results, these results are considered more reliable.

Conventional western medicine uses several parameters to measure the effectiveness of a treatment for hepatitis C:

- ○ Viral load becomes undetectable
- ○ Liver functions are restored

O Quality of life is improved

O The course of disease is slowed down or modified.

Evaluating hep C drug studies

When you read the results of a drug study, the first thing to keep in mind is that these studies are often conducted by the companies that make the drug. These companies want the success rates to be high, so that the drug will gain FDA approval, and of course they can make more money selling a drug that is supposed to be effective. This does not mean that the drug isn't effective. It just means you have to read between the lines, consult specialists, and do some research on your own.

Tips for learning about a drug's effectiveness

O Consult a variety of specialists, including doctors who are not involved in the study but are knowledgeable about the treatment.

O Since the drug won't be equally effective for all patients, find out which factors influence a patient's likelihood of responding to the drug.

As we mentioned above, studies show that the most effective drug for treating hepatitis C is a combination of **pegylated** (or time-release) **interferon** and **ribavirin.** The treatment is considered successful when HCV RNA is undetectable in a patient's blood six months following the end of treatment. According to some studies, the success rate is over 50 percent, but this varies according to a number of different factors—especially genotype. According to Schering-Plough, patients who received a combination of Peg-Intron and Rebetron had the following rates of sustained response:

O Genotype 2 had an 85 percent sustained response rate.

O Genotype 3 had 78 percent.

O Genotype 1 had 52 percent.[4]

Eighty percent of HCV-positive people in the United States have genotype 1. When you're evaluating a drug study, it's important to find out what percent of patients had type 1 and what percent had type 2 or 3. If the majority of patients had type 2 or 3, the overall success rate will be higher.

Factors that increase the likelihood of responding to combination therapy

- O Low viral load
- O Genotype 2 or 3, which are more likely to respond than 1 or 4
- O Short duration of infection
- O Infected with fewer strains of virus
- O Younger age
- O Healthy patient
- O Healthy liver
- O Female
- O Low iron levels. Menstruating women are more likely to respond than men because menstruation decreases iron levels. Once again, this is another reason for people with hep C to avoid iron supplements.
- O Low body fat.

One factor that greatly decreases the effectiveness of drug therapy is that many patients find it difficult to take their medications consistently, because the side effects can be so severe. Doctors have been working more closely with their patients to help them mitigate side effects and comply with treatment. For instance, a doctor might check on the patient's well-being and recommend therapy, acupuncture, antidepressants, or some other complementary treatment. This may seem obvious, but when patients take their medications, the medications work more effectively. A recent study shows that several factors increase the efficacy of interferon-ribavirin. These factors are:

- O How frequently the patients take their medication
- O How closely the medication is calibrated to the patient's weight.
- O How much of their medication patients take. The patient is prescribed a very precise dose of pegylated interferon, depending on his or her weight. The medication works mostly effectively when the patient takes all of it. But since interferon is injected, it's possible

not to take the whole dose at once. Some patients take partial doses to reduce the side effects.

When the medication is calibrated according to weight and patients take 80 percent of their medication 80 percent of the time, the success rate of interferon-ribavirin increases.[4]

Another important question to ask is how long the patients were followed after the end of treatment. Patients are classified as sustained responders if HCV RNA remains undetectable in their blood six months after treatment ends. Thus a 46 percent success rate means that 46 percent of the participants had no detectable viral load after 6 months. Studies have shown that most people who have no viral load six months after the end of treatment continue to have no viral load for up to six years following treatment.[5]

IN A SENTENCE:

> *At the moment, conventional western treatment consists of interferon-based therapies.*

FIRST-MONTH MILESTONE

By the end of your first month, you've taken steps to begin managing and balancing your daily life with hepatitis C:

○ YOU'VE MADE THE LIFESTYLE CHANGES YOU'VE SCHEDULED FOR THE FIRST MONTH.

○ YOU'VE GOTTEN HEALTH INSURANCE, OR CHECKED ON WHAT YOUR INSURANCE PLAN COVERS.

○ YOU'VE LEARNED THE SIGNS OF DEPRESSION AND HAVE SOUGHT HELP IF YOU THINK IT'S NECESSARY.

○ YOU'VE EXAMINED YOUR FAMILY PATTERNS OF DEALING WITH ILLNESS.

○ YOU'VE WORKED ON BUILDING YOUR SUPPORT NETWORK AND TALKED TO FAMILY AND FRIENDS ABOUT YOUR HEP C NEEDS.

○ YOU'VE LEARNED ABOUT CONVENTIONAL WESTERN TREATMENTS AND TALKED TO YOUR DOCTOR ABOUT YOUR TREATMENT OPTIONS.

Complementary and Alternative Treatments

AS WE discussed in Week 4, conventional western medicine for hep C concentrates on eliminating the virus through drug therapy and on replacing the liver if the patient will die otherwise. While western medicine focuses on very specific interventions, holistic approaches aim to treat the whole person. These treatments generally focus on restoring balance and boosting the body's natural defenses. Although holistic treatments are often called "alternative medicine," they don't have to be an alternative to western medicine. Many people use acupuncture and herbs to mitigate the side effects of interferon and other western therapies. For this reason, they are often called complementary treatments as well.

Many holistic treatments can be more subtle and less toxic than western pharmaceuticals. Unfortunately, most holistic treatments have not been studied widely—if at all—and the evidence supporting them is largely **anecdotal evidence**, meaning that it is based on the reports of individuals, rather than scientific studies. The fact that these treatments have not been widely studied does not necessarily mean that they are not effective or not safe. But, as with any treatment, you should consult a doctor or experienced practitioner before taking them.

Combining conventional and complementary treatments

○ You can combine Chinese medicine with western drug therapy, as long as you keep all your practitioners informed about what you're doing.

○ Acupuncture can be used in combination with any other treatment.

○ Don't combine herbal products you buy off the shelf.

○ Don't combine Chinese herbs with western or Ayurvedic herbs yourself. A herbalist may choose to combine them.

○ If you want to take herbs, definitely consult with an herbalist, rather than self-prescribing them.

○ Homeopathic and conventional "allopathic" treatments don't combine well.

We provide a brief introduction to traditional Chinese medicine, Ayurveda, and homeopathy in the Learning section of this chapter.

Many people with hep C take herbs

"Everyone in my support group recommended milk thistle. They told me to take milk thistle, so I bought a year's supply. It made my enzymes go down."

—JAKE O.

"I used to take any herbs that someone suggested to me. I would try anything. That was until my enzymes shot up into the hundreds. They had never been that high. My doctor asked if I had been drinking a lot. I told him about the herbs. He explained to me that just because it was natural didn't mean it was good for me. He used an analogy about poisonous berries. Now I think before I just take them."

—MYRNA H.

Many people with hepatitis C have turned to herbal therapies to relieve their symptoms as well as the side effects of interferon. Other people claim that herbs are dangerous because they're not regulated in the way medications are. This means we don't really know what's in the herbs we're taking. We suggest the following tips for taking herbs:

O Consult a Chinese or western herbalist. Reading about herbs is no substitute for expert advice, and it may be difficult to find accurate, reliable information about herbs that isn't written by people who are trying to sell you their product. Some good sources of information include:

- Blumenthal, Mark, ed. *The Complete German Commission E Monographs: Therapeutic Guide to Herbal Medicines.* Newton, MA: Integrative Medicine Communications, 1998.
- Blumenthal, Mark and Alicia Goldberg, eds. *Herbal Medicine: Expanded Commission E Monographs.* Newton, MA, 2000.
- Chevallier, Andrew. *Encyclopedia of Herbal Medicine: The Definitive Reference to 550 Herbs Common Ailments.* DK Adult, 2000.
- Fugh-Berman, Adriane, M.D. *Alternative Medicine: What Works.* William & Wilkins, 1997.
- Physicians Desk Reference Staff. *The PDR Family Guide to Natural Medicines and Healing Therapies.* New York: Ballantine, 2000.
- American Botanical Council
  www.herbalgram.org
- Herb Research Foundation
  303-449-2265
  www.herbs.org

O Try one herb at a time. Many formulations contain lots of herbs. This makes it harder to know what you're taking, how the different herbs are interacting, and what's working for you. Be sure to consult a specialist if you're thinking of combining herbs.

O Chinese, western, and Ayurvedic herbalism are three different systems of herbs, and they can't necessarily be combined. Chinese herbs in particular have to be prepared a certain way in order to produce the desired effect. As we said above, don't combine Chinese, western or

Ayurvedic herbs yourself. A herbalist may choose to combine them. We discuss Chinese medicine more in the Learning section of this chapter.

Unfortunately the effects of most herbs have not been studied. One of the major obstacles to studying herbs is that the ingredients of specific herbs can vary tremendously depending on the condition of the soil and how the plants are grown and harvested. Even if you're taking the same brand with the same label, you don't really know if the active ingredients are the same. This makes it difficult to study herbs and to compare the results of different studies. For more information on herbs, see Month 4 Learning

Milk thistle: The herb most commonly recommended for hep C

The medicinal properties of milk thistle have been touted at least since ancient Rome. Pliny the Elder (23–79 CE) said this herb's milky juice was excellent for "carrying off bile." The sixteenth-century British herbalist John Gerard prescribed milk thistle for "expelling melancholy," which was considered a malaise of the liver at that time. **Silymarin**, found in the fruit of the milk thistle plant, consists of silidianin, silicristin, and the most active ingredient, silybin. Although there is no evidence that milk thistle (Silybum marianum) cures hepatitis C, silybin protects the liver from the poisonous death cap mushroom (Amanita phalloides) and may be effective in treating liver disease as well.

In 2003, *The American Journal of Gastroenterology* published a systematic review of herbs used for treating hep C. Milk thistle was the only herb that demonstrated a significant decrease in liver enzymes in a **randomized double-blind placebo-controlled (RDBPC)** study.[1] The German government has approved milk thistle for treating hepatitis. But according to the National Center for Complementary and Alternative Medicine (NCCAM), this herb hasn't been studied enough, and the results of the few scientific studies are not sufficient from which to draw conclusions.

Studies in animals show that milk thistle may

O   help prevent liver damage by binding to receptor sites on liver cells and preventing toxins from entering

○ stimulate the growth of particular liver cells
○ act as an antioxidant, preventing free radicals from causing cell damage. Animal studies show that silymarin raises the amount of **glutathione peroxidase**, a powerful antioxidant that the liver produces. As an antioxidant, silymarin may have 10 times potency of vitamin E.[2]
○ inhibit liver inflammation.

How to take milk thistle

Since milk thistle does not easily dissolve in water, you can't get the benefits by munching the leaves or drinking it as a tea. It's best to take it in a capsule combined with an ingredient such as beta-cyclodextrin or phosphatidylcholine (silipede) that makes milk thistle more water-soluble. The *PDR for Herbal Medicines* recommends 200 to 400 mg of **silymarin** per day.[3] Try to get a standardized extract of 80 percent silymarin.

Possible side effects, allergies, and drug interactions

Milk thistle is probably safe, but some users report mild side effects, including diarrhea, headache, irritability, and nausea. Some people may have allergic reactions to milk thistle if they are allergic to plants of the same family, such as the chrysanthemum, daisy, marigold, and ragweed. Just as medications can interact with each other, medicinal herbs can interact with medications—increasing or canceling their effects. As with any herb or medication, it's important to tell your doctor and other health care providers if you are taking milk thistle.

Milk thistle may enhance the effects of the following medications and herbs:

○ methadone
○ antidepressants: bupropion (Wellbutrin/Zyban), paroxetine (Paxil), fluoxetine (Prozac), fluvoxetine (Luvox), nefazodone (Serzone), sertaline (Zoloft), and venlafaxine (Effexor)
○ St. John's wort, an herb taken for depression
○ antipsychotics: clozapine (Clozaril) and pimozide (Orap)
○ sedatives and sleeping pills such as zolpidem (Ambien), triazolam (Halcion), and midazolam (Versed)

○ Flecanide (Tambocor), propafenone (Rytrhmol) for heart conditions
○ antibiotics: erythromycin and rifampin
○ antiseizure medications: carbamazepine (Tegretol)
○ antihistamines: astemizole (Hismanal) and terfenadine (Seldane)
○ antifungals: itraconazole (Sporanox) and ketoconazole (Nizoral)
○ gastrointestinal motility drugs: cisapride (Propulsid)
○ ergot drugs: ergonovine and ergotamine (Ergbomar)
○ statins or lipid-lowering drugs: fluvastatin (Lescol), lovastatin (Mevacor), pravastatin (Pravachol), simvastatin (Zocor), cerivastatin (Baycol)
○ transplant drugs: as cyclosporine (Neoral, Sandimmune) and tacrolimus (Prograf).

Milk thistle may decrease the effects of the following medications:

○ sedatives/sleeping pills: lorazepam (Ativan)
○ hormones: estrogen
○ antiparasite drugs: atovaquone (Mepron)[4]

To learn more about the research on milk thistle, check the Web site of the National Institutes of Health's National Center for Complementary and Alternative Medicine (NCCAM): nccam.nih.gov/health/hepatitisc/. You can also contact them at:

National Center for Complementary and Alternative Medicine (NCCAM), National Institutes of Health
9000 Rockville Pike
Bethesda, Maryland 20892 USA
888-644-6226
Fax: 866-464-3616
www.nccam.nih.gov

Be sure to check with your doctor or licensed practitioner before you try any treatment, especially if you're taking herbs, which are powerful medicines. Many people think that because herbs are "natural," they're less potent than pharmaceutical drugs, but this is not always the case. If you want to take herbs, consult an herbalist. Don't self-prescribe. And if you're combining treatments, make sure all your health care practitioners know what you're doing. We'll come back to this topic in Month 4, where we provide lists of liver-friendly and liver-toxic herbs.

IN A SENTENCE:

> *Check with a doctor or experienced practitioner before you take or combine any treatments, medications, or herbs.*

learning

Traditional Chinese Medicine, Ayurveda, and Homeopathy

"I try everything I hear about to deal with my hep C. The thing I like best is acupuncture. Not only has it lowered my liver enzymes, but it is helping me quit smoking. After acupuncture I feel more centered, calm and much more clear. It is just one more thing that having hep C has opened me up to."

—VIOLET D.

"I have chronic hep B and C. I think I got them both at the same time, when I was between 16 and 19. I'm 51 now. I did Dr. Wei de Ren's Chinese herbal treatment 12 or 14 years ago. I didn't even know I had C then. I just knew I had B. When I started the treatment, I was so ill I couldn't get out of bed. I was treated for a year. I was in bed for the first three months, but after that my energy came back really fast. After the treatment, I felt better

*than I'd ever felt in my life. I've been pretty healthy since
then. Recently I had a flare-up, but it was because I worked
too hard taking care of my mother. A person with hepatitis
shouldn't work too hard or lose sleep."*

—SANDY W.

SO FAR we've talked about hepatitis C from the perspective of conventional western medicine. We've discussed a wide range of medical terms
and diagnostic tools, including *hepatitis, viruses, antibodies, antibody tests,
liver enzymes, liver functions,* and *biopsies.* All these terms and diagnostic
tools are derived from conventional western medicine, which understands
hepatitis C as a virus that attacks the liver. Traditional Chinese Medicine
does not recognize viruses and has no corresponding name for "hepatitis"
(meaning inflammation of the liver), although some CM practitioners study
western research on the HCV virus and use western diagnostic tools to
measure the progress of their patients. Some even specialize in treating
people diagnosed with hepatitis C.

Chinese medicine has been practiced for 3,000 years. It has recognized
and treated the symptoms of liver disease for thousands of years longer than
western medicine. Although the Cultural Revolution of the 1960s tried to
suppress Traditional Chinese Medicine, it is still the main form of medicine practiced in China.

Most people think of Chinese medicine as acupuncture. But Chinese
medicine is a much broader field that includes herbal treatments, nutrition,
meditation, massage and Qi Gong. If you're interested in being treated with
Chinese medicine, be sure to go to a licensed practitioner. You can take
classes or buy books, DVDs, and audiobooks on meditation and Qi Gong.

Chinese medicine: A more holistic approach

Chinese medicine is more holistic than conventional western medicine.
As we have discussed, the goal of conventional western medicine is to
eradicate the HCV virus, which it sees as the cause of disease. From a
Chinese medical perspective, it isn't so much the virus that causes illness
but rather the relationship between the virus and the person it infects.
Each person responds to the virus in a unique way and must be treated
individually.

Another difference between western and Chinese medicine is that western medicine tends to focus on the specialized tasks of one organ: For instance, according to western medicine, the liver processes nutrients and toxins and helps regulate the blood and sex hormones. Chinese medicine, on the other hand, sees these processes as a dynamic interaction of several organ systems—the liver organ system, spleen organ system, kidney organ system, and heart organ system. As mentioned above, Traditional Chinese Medicine has no concept of a "virus." It understands disease as an imbalance in the organ systems, and the liver is the "general" that keeps all the other systems in balance. Thus according to Chinese medicine, an imbalance in the liver organ system can throw other systems out of whack.

It's important to note, however, that this idea is not completely at odds with western medicine's understanding of hep C. Many western doctors understand and treat hep C as a systemic illness—a disease that affects the whole system, not just the liver. Although western medical doctors tend to specialize in one organ or part of the body, it would be a mistake to think that specialists, such as hepatologists and gastroenterologists, only know about the liver and stomach and intestines and won't understand how hep C affects the rest of you.

Nonetheless, western doctors are more likely to refer you to specialists in other fields. Another difference between Chinese and conventional western medicine is that Chinese medicine doesn't separate mind from body. The organ systems regulate emotions and mental states as well as physical conditions. The liver system regulates the emotions, so liver imbalance causes emotional upset, and emotional imbalance indicates liver disease. Thus a Chinese practitioner may treat depression, anxiety, and insomnia as part of an imbalance in your organ systems and make dietary recommendations, while a western doctor might refer you to a psychiatrist for depression and a nutritionist for dietary advice. It's never a bad idea to consult many specialists, but it can be frustrating, as well as expensive. This is one of the reasons why many people with hep C seek holistic treatments, such as Chinese medicine, as a complement or alternative to western medical care.

While Chinese medicine focuses on the whole person, some Chinese doctors, such as Misha Cohen, O.M.D., L.Ac., Wei de Ren, M.D., and Qincai Zhang, L.Ac., M.D., are especially committed to treating people with hep C. You can check out their Web sites for more information:

Misha Cohen, O.M.D., L.Ac.
www.docmisha.com

Wei de Ren, M.D.
www.dr-ren.com

Qincai Zhang, L.Ac., M.D.
www.dr-zhang.com

Misha Cohen coauthored *The Hepatitis C Help Book,* a program combining eastern and western treatments.

Ayurveda: Another holistic approach to healing

Ayurveda means "knowledge of life." Although much less commonly practiced in the United States than Chinese medicine, it is the national health care system of India and Sri Lanka. Practitioners treat people based on their dominant energies and body types. Recommendations include:

○ Detoxification
○ Yoga
○ Herbs
○ Nutrition
○ Meditation and prayer
○ Lifestyle changes.

Ayurvedic treatments are very individual. Therefore it's important to go to an experienced practitioner. You may want to get a reference from an Ayurvedic institute listed in the resource section. Ayurvedic herbs are also very powerful and don't necessarily mix well with other herbs and medications. Once again, check with all your practitioners before combining treatments.

Homeopathy

Homeopathy is the practice of treating an illness by giving the patient a tiny dose of a substance that produces effects similar to the symptoms of the disease. This contrasts with conventional western or "allopathic" medicine, which prescribes medications that produce effects different

from the disease. (*Homeo* means "same," while *allo* means "other.")
Homeopathic treatment is very specific to the individual, so you need to
see a practitioner who can prescribe medicine for you. Homeopathic and
allopathic treatments don't generally combine well. They are based on very
different principles.

Resources for complementary and alternative treatments

American Association of Oriental Medicine
PO Box 162340
Sacramento, CA 95816
866-455-7999
Fax: 916-443-4766
www.aaom.org

American Association of Naturopathic Physicians
4435 Wisconsin Ave NW Suite 403
Washington, DC 20016
Toll free: 866-538-2267
Local: 202-237-8150
Fax: 202-237-8152
www.naturopathic.org

HealthWorld Online
P.O. Box 1683
Sequel, CA 95073
www.healthy.net/herbalists

American Herbalists Guild
141 Nob Hill Road
Cheshire, CT 06410
203-272-6731
www.americanherbalistsguild.com

American Holistic Medical Association
PO Box 2016
Edmonds, WA 98020
425-967-0737
Fax: 425-771-9588
www.holisticmedicine.org

HealingPeople.com
Lists acupuncturists and healers across the country
www.healingpeople.com

Health Concerns
510-639-0280
Fax: 510-639-9140
www.HealthConcerns.com/pro

NCCAM, National Institutes of Health
9000 Rockville Pike
Bethesda, Maryland 20892 USA
888-644-6226
Fax: 866-464-3616
www.nccam.nih.gov
http://nccam.nih.gov/health/hepatitisc

National Certification Commission of Acupuncture
703-548-9004
www.nccaom.org

IN A SENTENCE:

> *Three popular alternative treatments for hep C include traditional Chinese medicine, Ayurveda, and homeopathy.*

living

Hep C Can Affect Your Long-Term Relationships

MANY OF us have partners, spouses, and friends who are supportive of us in our struggle with hep C. But sometimes hep C can threaten our long-term relationships.

Chances are your long-term partner won't get hep C from you through sex or through sharing household items. As we've mentioned before, if you have hep C and you're in a long-term monogamous relationship, your risk of transmitting it to your partner is 0 to 0.6 percent per year. Studies show that between 0 and 6 percent of the partners of hep C patients also have HCV. The average is 2 percent. If both you and your partner have hep C, chances are you didn't get it from one another unless you were doing IV drugs together. See Month 5 for more information about sexual transmission and talking to your partner about sex.

> *"Over the last year, my partner has gotten so tired he can hardly go to work. We just found out he has hep C, and I don't know if I can take it. I don't want to support him, and I'm afraid of watching him get sick."*
>
> —JANET Y.

*"When I got diagnosed with hep C,
my husband stopped having sex with me, and he can barely
touch me. He got tested and had the kids tested as well.
They're all negative, but I feel like an outcast."*

—KATIE R.

These situations are more common than you may think. Other messages we may hear or feel we're getting from our loved ones include:

- ○ I don't want to take care of you.
- ○ I don't want to hear about your illness all the time.
- ○ I don't want to support you financially.
- ○ I got hep C from you.
- ○ I gave hep C to you.
- ○ Who's going to support us if both of us get sick?
- ○ I'm afraid of getting hep C from you.
- ○ I'm afraid of giving hep C to you.
- ○ I feel as if you're dirty.
- ○ I feel too dirty to have sex.
- ○ I don't want to get pregnant and have kids with hep C.

If you're facing any of these issues, you're not alone. When we were diagnosed, we each wondered if we would ever find anyone who would want to have a long-term relationship with us. These fears were not completely unfounded. It isn't easy caring for a sick loved one. But it's important to put this in perspective: most people become chronically ill with some condition at some point in their lives, and most people with hepatitis C may never get seriously ill. And remember, if one of you gets sick, you can survive this. Sometimes dealing with illness can strengthen a relationship.

Check out the Well Spouse Foundation for more suggestions: www.wellspouse.com.

Since most long-term relationship issues are also day-to-day life issues, we've addressed many of them in other chapters.

- ○ Day 2 "Learning: Transmission: (especially "Use Standard Precautions")

○ Day 3 Living: "Telling People about Your Hep C" (especially "Telling Long-Term Partners and Spouses")
○ Week 2 Learning: "Insurance and Financial Planning"
○ Month 10 Living and Learning: "Children and Hep C" and "Teaching Kids About Hep C."

Even though the media is finally paying more attention to hep C, most people still know nothing about it and are quick to make assumptions. If you're in a long-term relationship and you talk about your own illness, people may assume your partner is also infected and treat him or her differently. It's a good idea to have open communication about whom you tell and whom you don't tell, or who knows and who doesn't. You never want to be in the position of telling someone your partner didn't want to tell. You also don't want your partner to be surprised that someone knows.

Unfortunately, sometimes an illness can cause partners to blame one another, especially if one of you gets sick or goes through treatment and has no energy for the relationship, work, or household responsibilities. Money may also become a sore point. It's important not to blame yourself or your partner for things you can't control. But this is easier to say than to do.

In many cases, when hep C threatens a relationship, this indicates a deeper rift, which may require counseling. You can refer to Month 8 for some tips for finding a therapist or support group. In the resource section, we offer references for counseling specific to hep C.

IN A SENTENCE:

> *Hep C may bring up difficult issues in many long-term relationships.*

learning

Trends in Research and Treatment

*"I've learned so much about medicine because of
my hep C. I used to like science in high school,
and it's totally renewed my interest."*

—JIMMY D.

THE CURRENT treatments for hep C leave much to be desired. People with genotype 1a, the most common type in the United States, take pegylated interferon and ribavirin for 48 weeks with possibly debilitating side effects and only a 50 percent sustained response rate. Moreover, sustained response is not the same thing as a cure. Patients are considered sustained responders when they have no detectable HCV RNA in their blood six months after completing treatment. But recent research has shown that the hep C virus continues to replicate in the livers of sustained responders—meaning that even if a patient has no HCV RNA in her blood, she may still have the virus in her liver and other organs.[1]

Nonetheless, this is a particularly promising and hopeful time for research on hepatitis C and the development of new medications. In 2004, scientists at the National Institute of

Diabetes and Digestive and Kidney Diseases (NIDDK) replicated HCV in a laboratory for the first time. They constructed a DNA copy of the HCV single-strand RNA genome and placed it into human liver cells in a cell culture medium. The replica behaved like a real hep C infection: It used the liver cells to produce copies of the virus, then released them from the host cell.[2] More recently, Nelson Fausto and his colleagues at the University of Washington produced a hep C virus culture system that allowed the virus to infect liver cells and produce new viruses that infected more liver cells for at least two months.[3] These culture systems represent major breakthroughs, allowing scientists to study the HCV virus's life cycle and to test potential antiviral medications.

In the following section we discuss the most promising new trend in hep C treatment, specifically, targeted antiviral therapy for HCV (or STAT-C), along with new developments in interferon and ribavirin, and therapeutic and preventative vaccines for hep C.

A new paradigm for hep C treatment: Specifically targeted antiviral therapy (STAT-C)

Recent scientific advances, including the culturing of HCV in the lab and the determination of the 3-D structure of parts of the HCV genome, have allowed researchers to develop and test antiviral molecules that target specific enzymes and parts of the virus that allow HCV to reproduce itself and infect new liver cells. This new class of drugs, specifically targeted antiviral therapy for HCV (or STAT-C), marks a major shift in the way hep C is treated. As we've discussed, the standard interferon-ribavirin therapy works by stimulating the immune system's response to the virus. Like the protease inhibitors used to treat HIV, the new STAT-C medications attack the HCV virus directly by blocking enzymes that the virus uses to replicate.

In a person with chronic hep C, one trillion HCV virions (replicated virus babies, so to speak) are produced per day. The life cycle of the HCV virus can be broken down into five stages. Medications that interrupt any step of this replication process could potentially be used for treating hep C.

O   Binding: The virus enters the liver cell through a receptor complex by a mechanism that is not fully understood. In the **cytoplasm** (the solution inside the cell surrounding the nucleus), the virus sheds its envelope and releases its single-stranded genome.

○ Translation: The virus takes over the host cell's **ribosome** (its protein-making machinery) and forces it to follow the virus's genetic instructions and make proteins that will be used to make new viruses. At this stage, the virus's RNA is translated into a polyprotein containing roughly 3,000 amino acids.

○ Protein processing: The virus uses **proteases** (enzymes or proteins that act as catalysts in biochemical reactions) to cut the polyprotein into smaller proteins in order to assemble a new virus. Theoretically, antiviral medications could be developed to target any of these viral proteins. Some of the drugs in development target the NS3 serine protease, which is produced during this stage.

○ Replication: Replication takes place in the replication complex. The proteins produced in the processing stage help duplicate the virus's genetic material—its RNA. The replication of the complete HCV genome depends upon a single enzyme: the HCV RNA-dependent RNA **polymerase**, which is produced during the protein processing stage. Some researchers are developing drugs called NS5B RNA-dependent RNA polymerase inhibitors that specifically target this enzyme.[4]

○ Assembly: Once the RNA is copied, it is used to make new infectious **virions**—individual particles of virus. Each new virion carries a copy of this RNA. The virions are finally released from the cell, so they can go infect other liver cells and start the process all over again. One hundred thousand virions can be released from one cell.

Theoretically, a drug that interrupted any one of these five stages could be used to treat hep C patients. The medications below are currently in clinical trials. It's important to remember that many of the drugs under development will never be FDA-approved because they will turn out to be ineffective or unsafe. One recent example is BILN 2061, a protease inhibitor made by Boehringer-Ingelheim that produced cardiac lesions in monkeys receiving large doses.

INTERNAL RIBOSOME ENTRY SITE (IRES) INHIBITORS

After HCV enters the cell and releases its genome (its RNA) into the cytoplasm, the virus recruits the host cell's protein-making machinery (called a ribosome) and forces the ribosome to follow the virus's genetic instructions (its messenger RNA) and make proteins that will be used to make new virions. This process is called translation, the second stage of the virus's life cycle. Researchers are developing and testing tiny molecules (appropriately named Internal Ribosome Entry Site Inhibitors) that interfere with the virus's internal ribosome entry site (IRES)—which makes translation possible. In translation, the ribosome has to be able to read the viral RNA correctly in order to assemble the proteins to make new virions. One kind of drug, called an antisense molecule, binds to the viral RNA and makes it unreadable. Another kind, a ribozyme, shreds the viral RNA. Two drugs have recently been tested in clinical trials: ISIS 14803, an antisense molecule, and Heptazyme, a ribozyme. Both have been discontinued because they were ineffective or toxic.

Nonetheless, IRES inhibitors represent a promising area of research, because they target a part of the HCV genome that remains the same throughout its mutations. As discussed above, HCV has a very high rate of mutation, which enables it to evade the immune system. Since a medication for treating HCV has to be effective against trillions of mutations, it is more likely to work if it targets a part of the virus's genetic material that does not mutate. The IRES is located on the 5' noncoding region—one of the few regions of the genome that tends to be copied correctly and conserved. By targeting the IRES, the antisense molecules and ribozymes "can't miss" the virus and are more likely to stop the virus from replicating.

PROTEASE INHIBITORS

Protease inhibitors are tiny molecules designed to target a specific site on an enzyme (or protease) and prevent that protease from performing its function in viral replication. Researchers are currently testing protease inhibitors that target the NS3 serine protease, which is produced in the protein processing stage. A number of protease inhibitors are in clinical trials, and some of them look especially promising for treating genotype 1a—the most common genotype in the United States—which is very resistant to the standard drug regimen of pegylated interferon and ribavirin. The protease inhibitors also seem more effective in treating African Americans and patients coinfected with HCV and HIV.

EXAMPLES OF PROTEASE INHIBITORS

Telaprevir (VX-950) is an oral protease inhibitor made by Vertex. According to a study by Henk Reesink and colleagues in the October 2006 issue of *Gastroenterology*, in a Phase Ib study telaprevir suppressed viral replication when genotype 1 patients took it alone or in combination with pegylated interferon for over 14 days. All 15 participants who initially received telaprevir, with or without pegylated interferon, and continued on standard therapy with pegylated interferon plus ribavirin had undetectable HCV after 24 weeks of follow-up.

In a separate study, 8 of 12 patients enrolled in a 28-day study of triple therapy with telaprevir, pegylated interferon, and ribavirin had undetectable HCV RNA after stopping telaprevir and continuing standard therapy for 24 weeks.[5]

SCH 503034, Schering-Plough's oral HCV protease inhibitor, is currently being tested in a large Phase II clinical trial on patients who did not respond to pegylated interferon and ribavirin. This drug has been fast-tracked by the FDA because looks promising in the treatment of non-responders with genotype 1a. SCH 503034 has shown potent antiviral activity and is well tolerated both as a monotherapy and in combination with PEG-INTRON and ribavirin.

ITMN-191, manufactured by InterMune, is a protease inhibitor that has not yet entered clinical trials. In an in vitro study, ITMN-191 in combination with pegylated interferon inhibited HCV replication at low concentrations of both drugs. On Dec. 19, 2006, they received the go-ahead to start Phase 1a clinical trials in Europe.

ACH-806 prevents the formation of the replicase complex

ACH-806 (AKA GS 9132), made by Achillion, prevents the formation of the replicase complex, a necessary step in viral replication that occurs after viral protein processing, the step that protease inhibitors affect, but before copying the viral RNA genome, the step that polymerase inhibitors affect. ACH-806 shows no cross-resistance to polymerase inhibitors or protease inhibitors, making it good to use in combination therapies. Based on Phase I, in-vitro testing, it appears to be as potent as Boehringer-Ingelheim's drug (BILN 2061), and 14 times more potent than the drugs being tested by Schering and Vertex.

POLYMERASE INHIBITORS

As mentioned above, the replication of the complete HCV genome depends upon a single enzyme: the HCV RNA-dependent RNA polymerase. Scientists are developing and testing HCV RNA-dependent RNA polymerase inhibitors that interfere with this enzyme and thus prevent the HCV virus from replicating itself.

EXAMPLES OF POLYMERASE INHIBITORS

Valopicitabine (NM283), an oral polymerase inhibitor made by Idenix Pharmaceuticals, has advanced furthest in this category. The phase 1b trial included 173 patients with genotype 1a who had never been treated before. (This is still considered a very small study.) After 24 weeks, doses as low as 200 mg/day markedly suppressed the virus in 68 percent of the patients, according to the report in October 2006. At higher doses, patients experienced gastrointestinal side effects.

R-1626 (Roche) Polymerase Inhibitor—This oral polymerase inhibitor will be used in conjunction with Pegasys and ribavirin (Copegasys) combination therapy. Phase I included 47 genotype 1 patients who received doses of 500, 1500, 3000 or 4500 mg or a placebo for 14 days. After the 14 days, the patients taking 3000 or 4500 mg showed dramatic reductions in HCV RNA. According to Dr. Stuart Roberts, these results were "the best that we have seen with all the polymerase inhibitors studied so far." There is about a 50 percent chance of success of a sustained viral response (showing no viral load six months after completing treatment) when used with combination therapy. Patients tolerated the R1626 relatively well up to doses of 3,000 mg but reported side effects at higher doses.

Experts say that in the near future STAT-C drugs will be used in combination with interferon and, in some cases, ribavirin. The addition of the new drugs may shorten the length of interferon-based therapy (which is presently 24 to 48 weeks) and consequently make this therapy less toxic. Eventually, patients may be taking "cocktails" of protease and polymerase inhibitors. A combination of drugs that attack the virus at different phases of its life cycle may be the best way to prevent the mutations that are resistant to treatment.

Innovations in interferon and ribavirin

ORAL INTERFERON

As we discussed, the alpha interferon used in treating hep C is a synthetically manufactured version of a protein that occurs naturally in the body. When infectious agents enter the body through the nose or mouth, the oral mucousal membranes produce interferon. Amarillo Biosciences, Inc. is trying to mimic this natural response by producing an interferon that patients can take orally at a much lower dose with fewer side effects. This interferon can be stored at room temperature, which will make it easier to take away from home.

ALBUFERON

Human Genome Sciences and Novartis are developing Albuferon, a long-acting interferon that may offer patients higher sustained response rates and a better quality of life. In clinical trials, subjects received injections of Albuferon every 14 days. When combined with ribavirin, Albuferon was as safe and effective as the other types of interferon, and it demonstrated greater antiviral activity than pegylated interferon. Patients reported fewer psychological side effects and did not have to take as many sick days.

INTERFERON IMPLANTS

The Omega Duros is a new delivery system rather than a new interferon. A tiny titanium tube is implanted under the skin and releases interferon gradually for up to three months. This device would probably make interferon-based therapy more effective because it eliminates the problem of patients forgetting to take their drugs. It would also make treatment much more convenient because patients wouldn't have to give themselves injections. They would simply visit the doctor a few times for new implants. Intarcia Therapeutics, the maker of Duros, has also developed a proprietary Omega interferon to use with their Duros system. So far, patients on Omega interferon combined with ribavirin have shown a favorable early sustained response rate (84 percent after 12 weeks). Long-term SVR data will be available soon.

RIBAVIRIN

As discussed in Week 4, many patients cannot take ribavirin due to debilitating side effects or medical conditions. Since ribavirin frequently causes hemolytic anemia, some people have to lower their dose or discontinue the drug altogether, and patients with preexisting hemolysis, anemia, or significant coronary or vascular diseases cannot take it. Patients with renal problems are also excluded from treatment due to the drug's potential effects on the kidneys.

Researchers have been trying to develop an alternative that has ribavirin's antiviral effects but doesn't cause anemia. The main obstacle is that no one understands how ribavirin fights viruses, or how it makes interferon more effective against hep C.

Valeant Pharmaceuticals is currently developing a safer alternative to ribavirin called Virmidine. In Phase III clinical trials, only 5 to 6 percent of the patients on Virmidine had developed hemolytic anemia, compared to ribavirin's 22 to 24 percent. Unfortunately, the patients on Virmidine also had lower sustained response rates: 40 percent, compared to ribavirin's 55 percent. Virmidine is now being tested at higher doses to see if the sustained response rate increases. Roche is developing a safer alternative to ribavirin, Levovirin, to be used with Pegasys.[6]

Vaccines

There is currenly no FDA-approved vaccine for hepatitis C, but some vaccines are in clinical trials. Most of these are therapeutic vaccines, rather than preventive vaccines. Preventive (or prophylactic) vaccines generally use weak or dead bacteria or virus to induce an immune response. The immune system remembers this immune response, so when the same kind of bacteria or virus invades, the immune system knows how to rid the body of the infection. A therapeutic vaccine, on the other hand, teaches the immune system to fight an existing infection. The purpose of a therapeutic vaccine is to reduce the infection's severity, or, ideally, to boost the immune system enough eliminate the infection.

While a therapeutic vaccine would help people already infected, a preventive vaccine would make life easier for everyone. It would stop the virus from spreading and reduce people's fear of transmitting or contracting hep C.

The only prophylactic vaccine currently in clinical trials is HCV/MF59 by Chiron/Novartis. One of the vaccine developers is Michael Houghton, who helped discover the hepatitis C virus. This vaccine combines sugary proteins derived from the surface of the virus with an oil-in-water emulsion meant to enhance the body's immune responses. For Phase II, CSL Ltd. and St. Louis University are testing humans with different doses of the vaccines and two different **adjuvants** (chemicals designed to help the body respond to the vaccine). The research is being sponsored by the National Institutes of Health and Chiron Corp. Early data from St. Louis University reported that 60 patients who received 4 different doses of vaccine all produced HCV antibodies.

The chief problem with the HCV/MF59 vaccine is that it works by getting the immune system to produce antibodies to HCV, and HCV can mutate rapidly and fool antibodies. Instead of antibody-mediated immunity, preventive vaccines may have to work through cell-mediated immunity, in which immune cells are taught to attack infected cells. Some of these vaccines are being developed, but they are all in preclinical phases.[7]

Other therapeutic vaccines in clinical trials

CHRONVAC-C/INOVIO BIOMEDICAL/PHASE I

This vaccine is designed to activate a T-cell response capable of clearing the hepatitis C virus.

PEVIPROTM/PEVION BIOTECT/PHASE I

This virosome-based vaccine for HCV uses synthetic peptide antigens from the hepatitis C virus. The vaccine helps the cellular immune response.

CGI 5005/GLOBEIMMUNE/PHASE I

This vaccine stimulates the immune system. Results from 40 patients found 3 patients had significant viral load reductions and a strong cellular immune response.

GV1001/Heptovax/Pharmexa/Phase II

Phase II has begun in Europe to treat liver cancer (HCC).

IC41/Intercell/Phase II

This is a combination of synthetic therapeutic vaccine, which increases the T-cell response, and peptides, identified through studies of people with natural immunity to HCV or a successful response to HCV therapy. Trials have shown reduction in viral load and T-cell response increase when used with pegylated interferon and ribavirin. A larger trial is planned for HCV genotype 1 patients.

INN0101 (E1)/Innogenetics/Phase II

Clinical trials are studying the effectiveness in slowing down fibrosis progression.

IN A SENTENCE:

> *Promising new treatments are being tested in clinical trials.*

Rebuilding Your Social Life Without Drugs and Alcohol

"I'm in my twenties, and I found out I have hep C. I used to go out to bars all the time with my friends and coworkers. Now I'm not sure what to do socially."

—Mona J.

"The hardest thing for me is not drinking. I am in college, and I feel really left out. Everyone around me drinks, and they wonder why I don't. I don't want to say I have hep C, because that makes me feel like a pariah. But I don't want to say anything else either. I just want to be part of the group."

—Darren O.

FOR THESE past three months, you may have put your social life on hold, while dealing with your diagnosis. Now as you enter Month 4, you may want to get back into the swing of things. Unfortunately, as you reenter your social world, you may find that some of your previous social activities are harmful to your health, especially if your social life included bars, cocktail parties, and three-martini power lunches. Cara realized that most of her friends hung out in bars, and she needed to make many changes in her social circle. Lisa never liked bars much, and liked them less after she was diagnosed with hep C, but she still finds it annoying that she can't drink on social occasions.

Since your liver processes most of what you eat, drink, breathe, and absorb through your skin, one of the best ways to take care of yourself is to avoid toxic substances. We've already mentioned the fact that alcohol and many recreational and prescription drugs are harmful to the liver. It's best to avoid them completely, especially if you have a substance abuse problem. Studies have shown that even moderate drinking can cause severe liver damage for people with hepatitis C, and our culture revolves so heavily around drinking that almost everyone with hep C will have to make lifestyle changes. If you have never used alcohol and drugs, or if you've been clean and sober for years, these issues may not apply to you, and you can go on to the next chapter. If you are only an occasional user, reducing your intake will most likely still be very helpful for you.

Addiction and 12-step programs

If you have an addiction, hopefully you have already begun making the lifestyle changes that you decided to make in Week 2. This chapter on rebuilding your social life goes hand in hand with making those changes. Many people find that AA, NA, and other 12-step programs help them rebuild their entire lives. When you're dealing with an addiction, it helps to hear how other people have gone through the same things. This common background and struggle can provide an immediate bond—the foundation of your support network. Twelve-step programs also sponsor parties, dances, and many other activities, which provide a safe space where you won't have to worry about being judged for having had an addiction, or for being clean and sober. These meetings and events can be a great venue for meeting new people, especially if all your friends use drugs and alcohol and you have a difficult time being around them.

Alcohol and your social life

Our culture associates drinking with having fun and being social. This is even more true in other cultures. When Lisa lived in Germany, no one understood why she wasn't drinking lots of beer. She told them about hep C, but some people still thought it was rude for a guest in their house not to drink anything.

Many people feel they need to drink to break down their inhibitions and have a good time. For some of us the hardest part of having hep C is giving up drinking as a way of relaxing and having fun. Alcohol is also a fake confidence booster, and it can give you an excuse for losing control and being wild. So when we give up alcohol, many of us feel as if we can't lose control anymore, and we don't have any excuse when we screw up. Dating is especially scary, and a lot of people start relationships by going out and drinking to ease the sexual tension and break the ice.

Unless you've made an effort to surround yourself with only clean and sober people, it's most likely going to be difficult for you to avoid being around alcohol. Almost everyone has friends, family, and coworkers who drink, and at least a part of their social life includes drinking. Some of you won't have a problem going to bars, parties, and restaurants, but for others this will be the hardest thing about having hep C. Those people need to find replacement activities and most likely look at their friendships. You can't ask other people to change their lives, but you can make friends who don't drink.

It may be hard to tell your friends that you can't drink, or do drugs anymore. Some people find it easier to tell people they have hep C than that they are recovering addicts. For suggestions on telling people that you have hep C, see Day 3.

> *"I used to be a junkie. I have been clean and sober for eight years. In the groups I hang out with, it's always been hard for me to explain why I don't drink. Two years ago I found out that I have hep C. I have a much easier time telling people that I have hep C than that I am clean and sober."*
>
> —TIM S.

Finding new friends and replacement activities

One of the best ways to make new friends and find people to date is to get involved in activities that don't involve alcohol and drugs. It's important to find things you love to do that help you let go and have fun. Take up an old dream or hobby, or begin something you've been dying to try for a long time. This is a good way to make friends who have common interests, and it will symbolize the fact that you're starting over and beginning a new phase of your life. Starting a new activity is also a good idea, because people tend to be supportive of beginners, and beginners can form bonds by growing together.

Many people use alcohol to break down their inhibitions and get out of their heads. But drinking is neither the healthiest nor the most effective way to quiet your mind or reach altered states. Some replacement activities include meditation, yoga, massage, Tai Chi, and exercise.

List 20 different activities you enjoy other than going to the bar, drinking, or doing drugs. For each activity, answer the following questions:

O What desires does it satisfy? What kind of fulfillment does it provide?
O Does it cost anything?
O Do you do it alone or with others?
O Does it have any health benefits?
O Is it dangerous?
O Can you do it easily on a regular basis?

Here are some examples:

O Going out to eat with different people
O Going on vacations or day trips
O Going out in nature
O Hiking and camping
O Taking long walks
O Having interesting conversations
O Going to movies, theater, concerts
O Exercising in groups, playing on teams, participating in sporting events

○ Taking classes you like, such as art or dance classes
○ Going dancing
○ Engaging in creative work
○ Overcoming artistic blocks. In *The Artist's Way,* Julia Cameron offers a book-length course in overcoming creative blocks.

> *"All of my relationships have started with some*
> *sort of drinking involved because alcohol makes it easier to*
> *break the ice. I asked one of my friends how he*
> *started relationships, and he said, 'I go out and get wasted,*
> *and then we end up in bed.'"*

—THERESA P.

Setting limits around our behavior

It's our responsibility to set limits around our own behavior. We need to figure out what we're comfortable with, and being at bars or around people who drink and do drugs might make us uncomfortable. It helps to hang out with people who respect your boundaries around drugs and alcohol and don't pressure you.

Exercise: Get moving!

Exercise is the best way to overcome an addiction. When you're addicted to any substance, especially opiates, your brain stops producing endorphins, because the drug takes their place. For this reason, you can experience a lot of depression and pain when you quit a drug. Exercise helps your brain begin producing endorphins again. It also relieves anxiety, stress, and muscle tension. It gives you more energy and helps you sleep. It also improves your circulation. This is especially important for former IV drug users, who may have damaged their veins.

Exercise can help you appreciate the benefits of giving up an addiction. When you give up an addiction, your body gets a lot stronger and your senses become more vivid. If you get outside, you'll enjoy the fresh air and sunshine more. You'll also be able to do more exercise, and this will show you how much healthier, stronger, and more confident you feel when you're not using.

Exercise can also be a good way to improve your social life, because you can join a gym or take classes. You can meet people through:

○ Yoga classes
○ Aerobics classes
○ Running, walking, or biking groups
○ Swim teams or other teams
○ Dancing.

> *"I used to get high from doing drugs. It's taken six years,
> but now I just exercise. I go out and run first thing
> every morning. The high is so much better,
> and I'm much happier."*
>
> —KAREN V.

IN A SENTENCE:

> *Having hep C can be a great impetus for building a social life
> without drugs and alcohol.*

Vitamins, Minerals, Herbs, Oh My!

THERE ARE vast amounts of literature on how vitamins, minerals, supplements, and herbs can help or harm people with hep C. Some of the material is trustworthy, but much of it is not. As you explore this material, the most important things to keep in mind are:

○ Find out as much as you can about any vitamins, supplements, or herbs you're thinking of taking
○ Consult your doctor before you take anything. It's even more important to ask your doctor before you combine a variety of products.

Vitamins and minerals: Too much of a good thing?

Vitamins and minerals are unlikely to hurt you if you take only the **Reference Daily Intake (RDI)**, formerly known as the **Recommended Daily Allowance (USRDA)**. Lots of research has gone into determining the minimum amounts of vitamins and minerals you need on a daily basis to avoid scurvy, rickets, and other vitamin and mineral deficiencies. If you eat a variety of fruits and vegetables, you're most likely getting enough vitamins and minerals.

The more controversial question is whether to take massive amounts of vitamins and minerals. Unfortunately, some substances that are good for you can kill you if you take too much of them. In the world of vitamins and minerals, you *can* get too much of a good thing. The fat-soluble vitamins (A, D, E, and K) are toxic in large quantities and accumulate in the liver. These substances are even more dangerous for those of us with hep C. We don't need any additional stress on our livers.

Liver-friendly vitamins and minerals

- B complex vitamins
- Vitamin C
- Vitamin E
- Selenium
- Zinc
- Calcium. This is especially important if you are avoiding dairy.
- Chromium
- Copper
- Folic acid
- Choline
- Inositol
- Iodine.

Vitamins and minerals that are good for you but toxic when taken in large amounts

- Vitamin A. Avoid supplements and multivitamins with high vitamin A content, especially more than 25,000 IU.
- Vitamin E. 400 to 1200 IU per day can boost your immune system, but don't take too much.
- Vitamin K
- Iron. Too much iron can be bad for people with hep C, especially for people with advanced stages of liver disease. Premenopausal women are less susceptible to this problem.

○ Selenium. Recommended dose is 100 mcg. More than 200 mcg per day can cause liver disease, hair loss, brittle nails, and bad breath.

"I had heard that drinking a glass of carrot juice a day was really good for people with hepatitis C. I thought that if carrot juice was good, then vitamin A must be good as well. I began taking vitamin A supplements and my liver enzymes shot up. I asked my doctor who told me there was a big difference in the way we got things like beta-carotene. He said that, yes, carrot juice was good, but that supplements were too much. From now on I'm going to consult a nutritionist and not self-prescribe."

—CARLOS R.

Do supplements work?

Most supplements have never been studied in clinical trials and are not FDA approved. This does not mean that they don't work. As we discussed in Week 4, clinical trials are typically sponsored by drug companies, and these companies have much more incentive to test profitable drugs than cheap ones. Many supplements, herbs, and other products that aren't produced by pharmaceutical companies will never get a chance to undergo clinical trials and obtain FDA approval. Once again, this is not because they don't work. It's simply because a drug company is unlikely to finance a clinical trial for a generic product or herb that any other company could then make and sell. In some countries, such as Germany, the government pays for clinical trials of herbs and other supplements. It would be to everyone's advantage if this were done here in the United States as well.

Nonetheless, supplements are not regulated in the same way medications are. This means that you don't really know what's in them. The actual ingredients may be different from what's on the label, and the ingredients can vary a lot depending on the brand.

If you're thinking of taking a supplement, the best thing you can do is read as much material as you can from different viewpoints—for and against. Read what conventional doctors have to say as well as what the supplement salespeople have to tell you. Remember, though, that salespeople may have different motivations than your health care provider. If the supplement has been studied, try to read the original studies. Don't trust everything you hear on the news, because many news reports are sensational and simplistic. Check Quackwatch (www.quackwatch.com), a Web site that warns consumers about scams.

If you do decide to take a supplement, be careful not to take too much. You can overdo supplements just as you can overdo vitamins and minerals. Some supplements can also interact with prescription drugs and cause adverse reactions. Some pharmacists know more about supplements than some doctors. So if you're taking supplements, it's not a bad idea to consult your pharmacist as well as your doctor. Let them both know all the drugs and supplements you're taking, and ask if there might be any contra-indications.

Liver-friendly supplements

○ Essential fatty acids. Flaxseed oil, linseed oil, evening primrose oil, raw sesame oil, and alpha lipoic acid can relieve joint pain and other aches associated with hep C and interferon treatment.
○ Colloidal minerals
○ SAM-e can relieve depression and may help protect the liver.
○ Wheat grass, chlorella, spirulina
○ Lecithin
○ Probiotics are living bacteria that can restore a healthy balance of bacteria in the intestines. *Lactobacillus acidophilus* is found in yogurt.

Liver-friendly amino acids

○ N-Acetyl-Cysteine (NAC). The body converts this supplement into glutathione, which plays a major role in the detoxification process.
○ Lysine is considered an antiviral.
○ Methionine helps the detoxification process.
○ Tryptophan can relieve insomnia, depression, and liver inflammation. It can be bought in the form of 5-htp.
○ Glycine also helps detoxification and reduces free radicals.
○ Glutamine and glutamic acid may protect the liver.

How about herbs?

The precautions concerning supplements apply to herbs as well. Many herbs haven't been studied. This doesn't mean they don't work, but it's crucial to learn as much about them as you can and ask your doctor before you take them.

Like other supplements, herbs are not regulated in the way medications are. As we discussed in Month 2, this means that you don't really know what's in them. The ingredients may vary tremendously depending on the condition of the source soil and how the plants are grown and harvested. Even if you're taking the same brand with the same label, you don't really know if the active ingredients are the same. This makes it extremely difficult to conduct studies on herbs and to compare the results of different studies.

Although the effectiveness of most herbs has not been scientifically studied, many people take herbs to alleviate symptoms of hep C and side effects of interferon. For some preliminary studies on alternative treatments, contact the National Institute of Health's National Center for Complementary and Alternative Medicine (NCCAM):

National Center for Complementary and Alternative Medicine (NCCAM), National Institutes of Health
9000 Rockville Pike
Bethesda, Maryland 20892 USA
888-644-6226
Fax: 866-464-3616
www.nccam.nih.gov

Liver-friendly herbs

O Astragalus is thought to promote immune function.
O Dandelion is used to treat liver disease.
O Milk thistle (*Silybum marianum*) is thought to protect the liver and is the most common herb taken by people with hep C. (See Month 2 Living for detailed discussion.)
O Schizandra also treats liver disease.
O Ginko Biloba is used for treating depression and memory loss.
O Licorice root
O Ginseng

○ Ginger
○ St. John's wort.

Practitioners of Chinese medicine use many combinations of herbs to treat liver disease. But once again, you need to see a licensed practitioner who can prescribe herbal formulations specifically designed for you. These formulations tend to vary from week to week or treatment to treatment.

Liver-toxic herbs

○ Plants of the Senecio, Crotalaria, and Heliotopium families
○ Kava Kava
○ Yohimbe
○ Valerian
○ Mate tea
○ Gordolobo yerba tea
○ Chaparral
○ Comfrey
○ Skullcap
○ Senna
○ Margosa oil
○ Pennyroyal oil
○ Germander
○ Asfetida
○ Mistletoe
○ Hops
○ Jin Bu Huan
○ Sassafras
○ Gentian
○ Groundsel
○ Ma huang (ephedra)
○ Nutmeg
○ Saw palmetto
○ Pau d'arco
○ Ragwort
○ Black cohosh
○ Buckthorn

This list is not exhaustive. Many other herbs can be toxic to your liver. It's best to check with an herbalist before taking anything. Don't self-prescribe herbs. See our tips for taking herbs in Month 2.

Resources

American Herbalists Guild
141 Nob Hill Road
Cheshire, CT 06410
203-272-6731
Fax: 203-272-8550
www.americanherbalistsguild.com

American Holistic Medical Association
PO Box 2016
Edmonds, WA 98020
425-967-0737
Fax: 425-771-9588
www.holisticmedicine.org

Health Concerns
510-639-0280
Fax: 510-639-9140
www.HealthConcerns.com/pro

Paths to Wholeness
Misha R. Cohen, OMD, L.A.c
415-861-1101
www.docmisha.com

Quan Yin Healing Arts Center
455 Valencia Street
San Francisco, CA 94103-3416
415-861-4964
www.quanyinhealingarts.com

IN A SENTENCE:

Consult your doctor and find out as much as you can about any vitamins, supplements, or herbs you're thinking of taking.

living

Yes,
You Can Have Sex!

*"The first time I had sex with my new boyfriend,
the condom broke. He knew I had hep C,
but we hadn't discussed the probability of sexual
transmission. He got onto MEDLINE and started
looking up every study he could find about the risk
of sexual transmission. After that I got the idea of
giving my sexual partners phone numbers they
could call to get information about hep C and the
likelihood of sexual transmission."*

—PAT M.

DON'T WORRY, you can still have sex. Hepatitis C is not
considered a sexually transmitted disease (**STD**), because it is
not primarily transmitted through sexual contact. In fact, hepatitis C has a very low risk of transmission through most forms
of sexual activity. According to experts from the Mayo Clinic,
if you're in a long-term monogamous relationship and your partner has hep C, your risk is 0 to 0.6 percent per year. If you're
in a short-term relationship with someone who has hep C, your

risk is 1 percent per year, and the CDC recommends routine condom use. This risk increases if your partner is HIV positive.

There are long-term relationships in which both partners test positive for HCV, but they might not have gotten it from each other. Studies show that between 0 and 6 percent of the partners of hep C patients also have HCV. The average is 2 percent. But it's not certain that these people contracted the virus from their partners through sex, since people in long-term relationships often have similar lifestyles and common experiences. Hepatitis C cannot be transmitted through hugging, kissing, or oral sex. Studies have failed to detect the presence of HCV in saliva, semen, or urine.

When we're talking about sexual transmission, it's important to define what we mean by "sex." A lot of people equate "sex" with heterosexual intercourse (a penis penetrating a vagina), but this definition excludes sexual activity between same-sex partners, oral sex, anal sex, masturbation, BDSM (bondage, discipline, sadism, and masochism), fetishes—in short, a virtually limitless array of erotic possibilities and alternative lifestyles. Basically anything a person eroticizes is a kind of sex for that person. So when we talk about how a disease can be sexually transmitted, it's important to recognize that there are many kinds of sex. HIV educators have acknowledged this for a long time, by drawing charts in which they break sexual activity down into "high risk," "low risk," and "no risk" behaviors. High risk for HIV includes unprotected anal and vaginal sex. Low risk includes unprotected oral sex, and no risk includes masturbation, foreplay, and kissing.

It's helpful to break down the risks for hep C in a similar way. High-risk behaviors would be those that provide a direct route from one person's bloodstream into another's. Most sexual activity does not involve this kind of direct blood-to-blood contact. In this sense, most sexual behavior is low risk. Nonetheless, the following activities and conditions pose a higher risk of blood-to-blood contact—hence a higher risk of HCV:

- Unprotected anal, vaginal, or oral sex when one or both partners have open lesions or sores, such as herpes blisters. Unprotected anal sex is especially risky because the lining of the anus tears easily. This is why it's relatively high risk for hep C as well as HIV.
- Unprotected vaginal or oral sex when one partner is menstruating
- Biting and breaking skin

○ Sores or cuts on the lips or mouth, bleeding gums. Try not to brush or floss your teeth right before sex, because brushing can make your gums bleed.

These factors increase the risk of hep C transmission. But you can greatly reduce the risk in any of these activities by practicing safer sex.

○ Don't let blood, semen, or vaginal fluids get into your bloodstream or come in contact with your mucous membranes.
○ Use latex or vinyl barriers such as condoms, dental dams, Saran Wrap®, and gloves.
○ If you use sex toys such as dildos or butt plugs, be sure to cover them in condoms and change the condoms before you use them on a different person. If there's a possibility that the toy might come in contact with someone's blood, you can cover the entire toy by putting a condom on each end.

As we said above, the rate of sexual transmission between long-term partners is very low. When you practice safer sex, the risk is even lower. Sexual activities that pose no risk of transmitting hep C include those that don't expose you to someone else's blood or body fluids—masturbation, hugging, and other casual contact. Kissing is also extremely low risk, especially when there are no open cuts or sores in your mouths.

Hep C prevention requires slightly different safer sex practices than HIV prevention. While the HIV virus "dies" almost immediately when exposed to air, the hep C virus can remain viable outside of the body for up to four days.

How is this relevant to sex? As we recall, sharing household items such as razors, toothbrushes, and manicure scissors poses a potential risk, because these items break skin. Thus, you can expose yourself to someone else's blood simply by using their razor. As we mentioned earlier, for many people, "sex" is not limited to intercourse, oral sex, or anal sex. There are people from various alternative lifestyles who use a wide range of equipment in their erotic play, and some of this equipment can break skin. Some examples are needles used for piercing, whips, hairbrushes, and anything with bristles or sharp points, can also break skin and draw blood.

It's important to know this in advance, because you may not even notice that you've drawn blood until after you've finished playing, and it's too late.

The best way to minimize the risk of transmission is to set boundaries for yourself ahead of time and to discuss these boundaries with your partner. It's up to each of us to decide which risks are acceptable and which are not. For instance, if you're a woman with hep C and you menstruate, you'll have to consider what precautions you want to take when you're on your period. Some of your options include:

- Using latex barriers for vaginal penetration and cunnilingus while you have your period
- Having some other kind of sex, but avoiding contact between your partner's mucous membranes and your blood
- Giving your partner information about hep C transmission and leaving it up to him or her to decide
- Not having any sex during your period.

It's good to decide your boundaries ahead of time, when you're in a sober frame of mind, and not in the heat of the moment. As many of us know, when we're turned on, we tend to do things we wouldn't otherwise do. But if we set limits beforehand, we're more likely to stay within them. It's also easier to stay within our limits when we don't mix sex with drugs or alcohol.

IN A SENTENCE:

The risk of sexual transmission is very low.

learning

Talking to Dates and Sexual Partners

OUR BOUNDARIES will be different with different people. What we're willing to do with a one night stand is not the same as what we're willing to do with a partner of 10 or 20 years. Just as it's important to decide your limits for yourself ahead of time, it's also important to negotiate with your partner ahead of time and decide what the two of you will and will not do. Communication is key! If you want to practice safer sex, be sure you're partner knows what you mean by safer sex. Some people are happy to wrap themselves head to toe in Saran Wrap®, while others won't even think of using a condom. For some people safer sex means oral sex with latex barriers; for others it doesn't. Clear communication can help you avoid unwanted pregnancy, STDs, and embarrassing situations.

Many of us wonder how we're going to tell future sexual partners about hepatitis C. We worry that they'll reject us. This fear can be especially strong for people who have just been diagnosed. When we were first diagnosed, we thought we'd never have sex again in our lives. This certainly doesn't have to be the case, although both of us have experienced a wide range of reactions. In our experience, a person's reactions provide a good indication of whether the relationship has a future or not.

It's understandable that your sexual partners may have concerns. You can allay their worries by providing them with some information, such as a hotline number or the URL of a good hep C Web site. See the Resources section in the back of the book.

Since the risk of sexual transmission is very low—and can be further reduced by practicing safer sex—it's likely that most people who want to have sex with you will still want to when they find out you have hep C. Give your partner time to process the information. If he or she can't get past the fear or even listen to the information, you may be better off finding a more supportive partner. Even if this is painful in the short term, you will both be happier in the long run.

When and how do you bring it up?

If you're planning to tell a potential sexual partner that you have hep C, we suggest you tell him or her before you have sex, rather than after especially if you're going to have unprotected sex, or engage in a relatively high-risk sexual behavior. Although there's very little risk involved in safer sex, most people like to be informed and have choices.

This may seem obvious, but it's also a bad idea to tell your partner that you have hep C right in the middle of sex. Tell them in a neutral setting.

The question is whom do you tell? For instance, do you tell your one-night stand? This is a tricky question. On the one hand, we have a responsibility not to infect others knowingly. On the other hand, a lot of sexual activity is very low risk, especially if you're practicing safer sex, which we recommend you do with everyone unless you know their sexual history quite well. When deciding whether or not to tell a casual partner, consider these factors:

- What risks are involved? Do you have your period? Do you have open cuts or sores?
- Are you going to feel anxiety or guilt later because you didn't tell the person? Guilt can manifest itself in a number of different ways. It's important to learn to recognize it.

O Are you going to see them again? If you think there's a chance you might have a relationship or friendship with them, you're probably going to tell them at some point, and they might be angry that you didn't tell them earlier.

If you do decide to tell someone—whether the first time or later—be prepared for a wide range of possible reactions.

O Some people will want to know about the risks, and once they find out that sex is low risk, they won't care.
O Some people might not know about hep C at all and need to be informed about the risks.
O Some people—hopefully not many—may have strong reactions and may not want to have sex with you.

"Stan was in town for a weekend on a business trip. I told him about my hep C soon after I first met him. He seemed fine with it, and after spending two nights hanging out together we ended up back at his hotel room. We began fooling around. I was shocked when he suddenly stopped and begged off, claiming he was too tired. The next morning he jumped out of bed and quickly dressed. I asked him what was wrong, and he told me that he was scared of contracting hep C from me. I had told him how low the risks were the night before, but he obviously didn't believe me."

—OLIVIA J.

"When I found out I had hep C, I had been in a long-term relationship for 13 years. Fortunately, my partner doesn't have it. We asked if we should start having protected sex. The doctor said that it was really low risk, and we should just keep doing what we were doing."

—FRANK MILES

We hope you'll have positive experiences telling your sexual partners about your hep C. Neither of us has ever regretted telling anyone. For the most part people have been understanding and accepting. When they weren't, we were better off not having them in our lives.

Review of safety precautions:

- ○ Avoid all blood-to-blood contact.
- ○ Don't share razors, toothbrushes, or anything that draws blood.
- ○ The virus can live for up to four days on razors and other objects (including various kinds of toys and equipment used in sex play), that may have come in contact with an infected person's blood.
- ○ Avoid contact between menstrual blood and sores, cuts, or mucous membranes.
- ○ Avoid contact between open wounds—especially on your hands, mouth, or genitals—and sores, cuts, or mucous membranes.
- ○ Use condoms.

> *"Five years ago, my new girlfriend bit me and accidentally drew blood. Afterward I told her that I had hep C. She said she had hep C too. She said she would have liked it if I had told her that I had it, but then she realized she didn't tell me she had it either."*
>
> —LISA M.

IN A SENTENCE:

> *Talk to your sexual partners and avoid blood-to-blood contact.*

MONTH 6

living

The Stigmas
Surrounding Hep C

*"I'm already so ashamed of being a junkie.
Now I have hep C, and I feel as if that
announces to everybody that I'm a junkie."*

—MARCUS R.

*"In my hep C support group, people would talk
about how they got the disease. There was this
hierarchy in which people who got the disease
through transfusions were 'good people,' and people
who got the disease through drugs were the 'bad
people,' who 'deserved' hep C. I don't know how I
got the disease. I've never done drugs, and people
called me a liar. We all have this disease, and we
need to focus on what we can do about it, instead
of bickering about which of us deserve it! Nobody
deserves hep C—no matter what they've done."*

—JANICE H.

*"I am a successful guy. I have a great, well-paying job as a
consultant. I am married with two kids. I have everything I've
always wanted. I also have hep C. I messed around with
drugs once or twice when I was younger. I wish I hadn't.
Usually I lie about how I contracted hep C.
I say I don't know. I still feel like people are suspicious of me.
As if I don't deserve everything I have now."*

—BART M.

It's important to debunk several myths that are damaging to people with
hep C.

○ Hep C is commonly transmitted through sex.
○ People with hep C are IV drug users.
○ People with hep C are contaminated and dirty.
○ People with hep C have lived a debauched lifestyle, including
promiscuous sex, as well as drug use. This is a version of the myth
that disease is the result of sin or moral decay.

Many people believe that hep C is primarily transmitted through sex.
Unfortunately, the media often reinforces this myth. We have seen this in
glossy magazines and newspapers and heard it on radio and TV news. As
we discussed in the last chapter, sex is a very inefficient means of transmission. It's important to question information you read or hear in the
media and check it against a reputable source.

You can show people statistics on the low rate of sexual transmission,
but some people see hep C as a sign of being debauched, dirty, or diseased.
This is much harder to refute.

Many of us have also encountered the assumption that because we have
hep C, we must have done IV drugs. Whether or not we've done drugs, we
don't deserve this stigma.

Although HCV can be transmitted by sharing needles and other "works,"
this accounts for only a small proportion of the HCV infections worldwide.
However, as we discussed in Day 2, IV drug use is only the primary route
of transmission in industrialized nations, where medical procedures are
usually performed with sterilized instruments under sterile conditions.
From a global perspective, the use of contaminated medical equipment is

by far the most common means of transmission. Three hundred million people worldwide have been exposed to hepatitis C. The vast majority of these people were not exposed through IV drug use. This myth is damaging to everyone.

Ironically, much of the silence and stigma around hepatitis C stems from the myth that IV drug use is the main method of transmission. Those of us who have never done IV drugs may find that our friends, family, or health professionals assume we contracted hep C through IV drug use and treat us differently as a result. But however you got this disease, you deserve the most up-to-date information, the best health care, and the best support possible.

Occasionally you may hear someone say that IV drug use "causes" hep C, in the same way that some people say alcohol "causes" hep C. This is false. IV drug use can put you at risk for hep C, but it doesn't "cause" hepatitis C. The causal agent is a virus that can enter the bloodstream through any behavior or situation that allows for blood-to-blood contact. As we learned in Day 2, the rate of transmission through shared needles and blood transfusions is high, but the rate of transmission through sex is considered low, as long as the sexual activity doesn't involve blood-to-blood contact. We don't need to avoid sharing utensils, hugging, kissing, or most kinds of sexual activity.

"I began a relationship with a friend I had known for a long time. The day after we had sex he told me that all of our friends had called him and given him a hard time about my hep C. They asked him if he was scared of contracting it and asked him what he was doing and if he was crazy. I had explained the low rate of sexual transmission to him but he still felt awkward and unsure after having to explain this to all of our friends. They stigmatized him just because he was with me. I felt horrible and embarrassed."

—CASSIE G.

It's important to understand that the stigmas surrounding hep C result from ignorance. People just don't know about hep C. When many people hear the word "epidemic," the first thing they think of is AIDS or **HIV**. Although HIV is more lethal, hep C is far more widespread: HIV has infected 40.3 million people worldwide. Three hundred million have hep C. Due to lack of public awareness, the specters and stigmas of AIDS overshadow hep C. Some people think these two viruses are almost the same. People need more accurate information about both HIV and hep C, so that they can protect themselves against both.

As people with hep C, many of us have faced stigmas similar to those of HIV. In the early 80s, AIDS was called a disease of "homosexuals, heroin addicts, and Haitians," as if it only affected a small, marginalized portion of the population. Similarly, when the media first began to talk about hepatitis C, it called it a "junkie disease." This misled some people into thinking: "It's not my problem. I don't know anyone who has this disease. The people who get it are the outsiders who screw themselves up anyway." This is patently false—as well as deadly. The truth is that people from all walks of life—including one's friends, family members, and oneself—could be infected with HCV. Finally the media is beginning to realize that hep C affects everyone. The more the media portrays hep C as a mainstream problem, the more likely we are to get government funding for research and treatment.

> *"I have been reading a lot about getting tattoos and how dangerous they are. I read one article about how a lot of people with tattoos also have hepatitis C. I'm wondering if people with tattoos are just more likely to engage in other 'alternative' acts like experimenting with drugs or if tattooing is really a risk. Aren't places required by law to be clean?"*
>
> —BEN S.

Until recently, tattooing was considered a risk, but tattooing is only dangerous when it is done with nonsterile equipment. You should never assume that someone has hep C just because they have tattoos.

Examining how hep C has affected your self-image

Many of us find that the stigmas surrounding hep C can affect our self-image. The first step is to be aware of when and how this happens. Consider the following questions:

O Do you feel as if some people treated you differently when they found out that you have hep C?

O How have your doctors treated you? How do you feel about it? How do you expect people to react when you tell them you have hep C?

O How have different people reacted?

O Have they met your expectations or surprised you?

O How has having hep C affected your self-image?

O If you contracted hep C through sharing needles or some other type of stigmatized behavior, do you find yourself having a lot of regrets about what you did? If so, start writing about what you regret and what you're thankful for. Begin by writing down all your regrets, then write down the positive things that have come out of your hep C infection. We may, for instance, regret sharing needles or having tried IV drugs in the first place. But perhaps the blessing is that we got clean. Some of us are thankful that hep C is the only "negative result" of our drug history.

Many of us can't help the fact that having hep C will affect our self-image to some extent. We can't change other people's reactions, but we can control how we take care of ourselves by choosing whom we tell and trying to surround ourselves with supportive people. If you feel like an outcast, going to support groups may help remind you that you are not alone.

IN A SENTENCE:

> *We can't change our past, but we can control our attitudes about it and change the way we interpret it.*

learning

Protecting Your Rights at the Workplace and Your Medical Records

"I had been working at my job for almost five years. Someone found out that I had hep C and told everyone. Suddenly, people began treating me like I was a leper. They whispered behind my back constantly. My boss must have found out as well, because she stopped giving me good assignments. I feel like she wants me to quit."

—Nancy G.

"My hep C sometimes leaves me so fatigued I can't work. I work construction. I told my boss, and he said that he felt bad for me but that if I was so tired maybe I should consider only working part-time or getting a job that didn't require physical labor. What am I going to do?"

—Chris W.

The Americans with Disabilities Act (ADA)

There are some situations in which hepatitis C might make it difficult for you to work. Some people experience bouts of acute hepatitis with severe flulike symptoms. Other people report prolonged debilitating fatigue, joint pain, or depression.

The Americans with Disabilities Act (ADA) makes it illegal for your employer to discriminate against you on the basis of a disability. You may not think of yourself as disabled, but the ADA may protect you if your employer fires you or turns you down because of a health condition, including a chronic illness like hep C.

According to the ADA, a physical or mental disability is a condition that restricts a major life activity such as seeing, walking, hearing, breathing, speaking, caring for oneself, learning, working or performing manual tasks. The ADA determines whether or not a person has a disability regardless of corrective measures, such as medications, hearing aids, prosthetic limbs, or other devices. People with chronic illnesses may be defined as disabled even if they are not sick all the time. If you have hep C and have intermittent bouts of illness, you may still be protected under the ADA.

Under the ADA, you cannot be discriminated against on the basis of hep C if you meet all the qualifications for your job, including work experience, education, skills, licenses, and any other requirements. You do not need to apply for federal disability insurance to be protected under ADA, but you do need a doctor's report that substantiates your disability.

How the ADA protects you at the workplace

- ◯ If you are ever fired or turned down for a job because of a health condition or the results of a medical exam, the employer must provide proof you are physically incapable of performing your job.
- ◯ Your employer must provide reasonable accommodations to make the workplace readily accessible for you and enable you to do your job.
- ◯ It is illegal for your employer to ask whether you are disabled or how severe your condition is.
- ◯ It is unlawful for a potential employer to require you to take a medical exam before you have been offered the job.

- Once your employer offers you the job, they can ask you to take a medical exam before you begin working—but only if it's mandatory for all employees.
- All medical records must be kept confidential and in separate files.
- The ADA does not cover anyone who is using illegal drugs. It is legal for your employer to give you a drug test, which is not considered a medical exam. Employees may be fired on the basis of drug use. The ADA does cover people who have completed a rehabilitation program.
- Your employer must give you access to the same benefits and privileges as employees without disabilities.
- Your employer must provide equal access to the same health insurance coverage that other employees have. The ADA does not require that your employer give you additional insurance coverage because of your condition. Your employer does not have to provide insurance that covers preexisting conditions.
- The ADA protects people with HIV disease.
- Your employer must post a notice explaining ADA requirements.

If you believe you've been discriminated against

Within 180 days of the discrimination, you may file a charge of discrimination at a local office of the U.S. Equal Employment Opportunity Commission (EEOC). In some states you have 300 days to file a charge. When you file a charge, it's important to bring a report from your doctor saying that you're disabled. You can look in the U.S. Government section of the white pages of the phone book to find the number for the EEOC. You can also check online at www.eeoc.gov/types/ada.html.

*"I work in a very nondiscriminating environment
and feel very lucky because of it. There are people in my
hep C support group who have come out to their workplace
and now are looked at weird if they even sneeze.
I want to change jobs but am afraid based on the fact
that other people don't have it so easy."*

—AMANDA W.

*"No one at my work knew what hep C was.
I discovered that if I was going to tell them, I also needed to
become a hep C educator. I decided to tell them while
providing information. I not only feel more comfortable and
open at my workplace, but I have found that I enjoy teaching
people about hep C. It puts me more in touch and
more at ease with my own illness."*

—MARGARET S.

Medical rights

*"I got hep C shooting speed. When my doctor asked me,
I told him because I wanted to be honest.
Now I'm so worried that the fact that I was shooting speed
is on my medical records."*

—KEVIN A.

What are your medical records?

Whenever you see any health professional including a doctor, nurse, psychiatrist, dentist or chiropractor, they jot down notes on your symptoms, their observations, and the treatments that they prescribe for you. These notes may contain your laboratory results, prescribed medications, results of surgical operations or procedures, your medical history, family history, anything they observe about you, and anything you tell them about your lifestyle, such as whether you smoke or engage in high-risk activities.

Currently the laws protecting the privacy of your medical records vary from state to state. In many states, the law requires that your doctor keep your medical records confidential, but you usually have to partially waive this confidentiality in order to get insurance companies to issue you a policy or provide coverage.

How to protect your medical records

O When you're asked to sign a document, read it carefully, and don't be afraid to edit it.

For instance, when you visit your doctor, you may be handed a piece of paper asking you to sign a "blanket waiver." The blanket waiver usually reads:

"I authorize any physician, hospital or other medical provider to release to [the insurance company] any information regarding my medical history, symptoms, treatment, exam results or diagnosis."

You don't have to sign the blanket waiver as it is written. You can modify the waiver to restrict the amount of information released. Here's how you can edit the waiver:

"I authorize [X doctor or hospital] to release my records to [the insurer] for the [date] as it relates to the [condition treated]."

O When you're asked to fill out a medical questionnaire, find out the purpose of the questionnaire and who will have access to the information. Your insurance company may use the information to raise your premium. If you say you've been smoking for 20 years, you can expect to pay more. Find out if you have to answer the questions or if you can do it anonymously.

O Your medical records become public record if they are subpoenaed for a court case. If you ask the court to restrict the records that are used as evidence in the case, a judge will determine what parts of your record can be kept private. After the case, you can request that the judge seal the court records that include information about your medical history.

Some communication technology may not offer much privacy

O Due to the U.S. Patriot Act, the privacy of U.S. postal mail is no longer protected by law. E-mail and fax transmissions are even less private. In a lot of offices, anyone can pick up a fax transmission. Your employer has the legal right to read all e-mail that you send or receive from your work computer or work e-mail program. If you do not want your employer knowing about your hepatitis C, you should not mention it in e-mails from work.

O Cordless and cellular telephones transmit radio waves that can be picked up by some electronic devices. If you want a conversation to be completely private, you're safest using a land line.

O Any information you disclose on Usenet chat rooms or newsgroups is easy to access. To protect yourself, don't register your name on Web sites. Use a pseudonym, or set up an account with Hotmail or Yahoo!, which don't require you to give your real name.

HIPAA

In the insurance section, we discussed HIPAA (Health Insurance Portability Accountability Act). There are two parts to HIPAA: the insurance provisions and the privacy provisions. Under privacy, the Administrative Simplification (AS) provisions require the establishment of national standards of health care transactions and security and privacy of data. The Privacy Rule (April 2003) establishes regulations for use and disclosure of patients' health information, including medical records and bill payments.

Getting copies of your medical records

Most clinics and doctors' offices will provide copies of your medical records, if you make a request in writing and pay a small fee. Lisa has obtained copies of her medical records that were seven or eight years old. In some cases, you may have to fill out a special release form. The laws surrounding medical records vary from state to state. Some states demand that doctors give you your records immediately, while others consider the records property of the hospital or medical establishment, rather than *your* property. In some states, doctors and clinics can discard medical records after a certain period of time has elapsed. If your records have been discarded, there is not much you can do.

There are a few simple steps to make getting your medical records easier:

○ If you have to make a request in writing, find out the person or agency to whom you should address this request.

○ Find out if you need to send payment, have your request notarized, or meet any other special criteria. You may even want to send a certified letter to make sure your request arrives and to have evidence that you sent it.

○ Send a brief letter stating exactly what you are looking for. Be sure to say that you are requesting copies of your own records and that you're over 18. Include your full name, birthdate, Social Security number, and the dates you received treatment. If you've changed your name, mention it. If you would like your records sent to another doctor, give his or her name and address as well. Sign your request, and include your phone number, address, and e-mail address, if you have one.

○ If they deny you access, ask for a written letter of denial.

The Medical Information Bureau (MIB) is a database containing files of medical information on 15 million American and Canadians. If they have a file on you, you can request a copy by contacting them. The first copy is free. You may contact them by calling 866-692-6901 or online at www.mib.com.

IN A SENTENCE:

> *As a person with a chronic illness, it is vital that you know your rights and keep copies of your medical records.*

HALF-YEAR MILESTONE

Now that you're halfway through your first year with hepatitis C:

○ YOU'VE LEARNED ABOUT ALTERNATIVE TREATMENTS.

○ YOU'VE CONTINUED TO MAKE THE LIFESTYLE CHANGES YOU NEED TO MAKE.

○ YOU'VE RESEARCHED AND ASKED YOUR DOCTOR ABOUT ANY VITAMINS, MINERALS, SUPPLEMENTS, AND/OR HERBS THAT YOU'RE INTERESTED IN TAKING.

○ YOU'VE LEARNED SKILLS FOR TALKING TO NEW AND LONG-TERM PARTNERS ABOUT HEP C.

○ YOU'VE TAKEN STEPS TO REBUILDING YOUR SOCIAL LIFE WITHOUT DRUGS AND ALCOHOL.

○ YOU'VE BECOME MORE CONSCIOUS OF THE STIGMA SURROUNDING HEP C.

○ YOU'VE LEARNED YOUR RIGHTS IN THE WORKPLACE.

○ You've ordered copies of your medical records, if you don't already have them.

As you now enter the last half of the year, you can expect to adjust to living with hep C, and:

○ Learn how to do research

○ Learn about the stages of liver disease

○ Learn about liver transplants

○ Get involved in hep C communities—locally, globally, or both

○ Learn about hep C issues specific to children

○ Learn about coinfection with HCV and other viruses

○ Review the past year and your accomplishments.

MONTH 7

living

Keeping Up to Date and Doing Research

NEW RESEARCH on hep C is constantly appearing in journals, newspapers, books, and on the Internet. You can find books with general information on hepatitis C in libraries, at the bookstore, or on online bookstores such as Amazon.com. One of the first things Cara did when she was diagnosed was a search for books on Amazon.com. Unless you have a background in medicine, we suggest that you start with these general information books, then move on to more specialized reading, such as articles in medical journals. This is what we did. We provide a list of both general and specialized resources in the "Further Reading" section.

Keep in mind that Amazon.com does not give an exhaustive list of the books out there, and public libraries may have an even more limited selection of hep C resources, unless you go to really large public libraries, like the main branch of the New York Public Library in New York City. If you are looking for more specialized information, such as scientific studies, you are better off looking in a medical library at a local hospital or medical school. You can find some medical journals at a college or university library as well. Some, such as *Hepatology,* are even available on the Internet, as we discuss below.

The World Wide Web

If you're researching a new treatment or study, you'll want to look on the World Wide Web. The Web is easily accessible from your home. Many sites on the Internet are updated daily. This is an excellent source for breaking news. Some medical and scientific papers are often posted and summarized in news articles. You can find almost any major news source online. You can also find many back issues and archives of newspapers. For instance, you can go to the *New York Times* Web site (www.nyt.com), click on "archives," look up every article on hepatitis C that has published in the last five years, and buy copies of the ones you want. To go directly to the archives, type in: http://search.nytimes.com/search/.

There are hundreds of Web sites devoted solely to hepatitis C, and a recent search on Google produced millions of page references to hep C. Search engines, such as Google, Yahoo! and Alta Vista, can help you find information on the Internet.

The Internet contains vast amounts of information, and much of it is not very structured. Search engines are pretty random: They do not necessarily pull things up in the order of importance, relevance, or ease of comprehension. Usually you have to wade through many Web sites to find what you want. Many sites, such as MEDLINEplus, offer well-organized databases, but there are just as many, if not more, that are poorly structured. Keep in mind that your first result may not be the best, and just because someone put up a Web page doesn't mean that the information on that page is accurate. Sometimes it's downright false. It's important to get information from reliable sources—-especially when your health is at stake.

Where can I find answers to my health questions?

MEDLINEplus, a service of the National Library of Medicine (NLM), provides information about various health conditions and diseases. The site also contains links to multilingual medical dictionaries, various hospitals, doctors, and clinical trials. The URL is www.nlm.nih.gov/medlineplus/.

For information on clinical trials, go to www.clinicaltrials.com and www.centerwatch.com. For the most up-to-date information on which drugs have been approved by the FDA, go to www.fda.gov/cder/da/da.htm.

For questions about complementary and alternative treatments, go to Ask Dr. Weil: www.drweil.com. Misha Cohen's site: www.docmisha.com is an excellent source of information on Chinese medicine and hepatitis C.

Where can I find explanations of scientific terms?

As you read more about hep C, you may come across scientific terms that you are unfamiliar with or would like to learn more about. If you're on MEDLINEplus, you can go to a medical dictionary. But the definitions you find in a medical dictionary may be too technical, and you might want something more basic. It helps to have a medical book and some biology textbooks, which you can borrow from your local public or university library. You can also consult an encyclopedia or reference book in print or on-line. Try the *Columbia Encyclopedia* or *Gray's Anatomy* at www.bartleby.com, or the *Encyclopedia Britannica* at www.britannica.com. How Stuff Works (www.howstuffworks.com) does not have the breadth of an encyclopedia, but it often provides much more thorough explanations of scientific phenomena. Ask Jeeves (www.askjeeves.com) can be great for finding news articles and textbook explanations.

If you want more specialized information, you can find some great academic search engines at www.academicinfo.net—the "'white pages' of the academic community." Once you're at the Academic Info Web site, you can click on topics like "biological sciences," "health and medicine," or "virology." This will take you to more specialized search engines and servers, which provide links to databases, journals, academic departments, scientists' Web sites, and more. Lisa uses Academic Info a lot, but when she's looking for medical articles, she prefers to search MEDLINE by medscape.com, as we explain below. This is one of the quickest and easiest ways to find medical articles on topics you're interested in.

Where can I find medical articles online?

The best place to search for medical articles online is MEDLINE, the database of the National Library of Medicine (NLM). MEDLINE contains information on more than 11 million articles from 4,300 biomedical journals. You type in the subject, author, or key words you're searching, and MEDLINE provides you with a list of articles on your topic. Sometimes MEDLINE gives only the author, the article's title, date, journal name and page numbers, but often it provides an abstract—that is, a brief summary of the article—or even the full article.

You can get free access to MEDLINE through the following sites:

www.medscape.com
www.ncbi.nlm.nih.gov/pubmed
www.pubmedcentral.nih.gov

Medscape.com is the most user-friendly. You can also go to the gastroenterology page, or the "resource center" for hepatitis C, at www.med scape.com/resource/hepc.

As mentioned above, MEDLINE doesn't always provide full articles on your subject. Sometimes it just gives bibliographical info or an abstract. If you want to read the full article, you might have to go to a medical library and look up the article in a journal. Some medical journals are available online. *Hepatology* is the journal of the American Association for the Study of Liver Diseases (AASLD). *Gastroenterology* (www.gastro jounal.org), the official journal of the American Gastroenterological Association requires a subscription fee. Hepatology Watch (www. hepwatch.com) provides brief summaries of breaking information for physicians.

Evaluating scientific studies

If you are not familiar with scientific studies and how they become published in medical journals, you may want to review "How New Medications Get on The Market" in the Learning section of Week 4. Basically, after a trial, the researchers write an article on the results and submit it to a medical journal. Before the journal publishes the paper, it may ask a group of "peers" (other researchers) to evaluate the research and decide whether it's fit for publication.

By the time something is published in a medical journal, experts have reviewed it. Some studies published in medical journals or summarized in newspapers are extremely reliable. But that does not necessarily mean that you should take everything they say as absolute truth. You shouldn't trust something just because it's science or published material.

Statistics are a good example of this. We all know people who will just quote statistics at us. Newspapers do this a lot. A good example is: "Forty percent of Americans take too much vitamin C." When you read a statistic like this, some of the questions you might want to ask are: What was the premise of the study? What was it trying to prove? What is the context? What group of Americans were studied? How were they chosen? How long were they studied? Was there a control group of people that weren't taking vitamin C? What amounts of vitamin C were taken? What is considered too much vitamin C? What is a safe amount of vitamin C? This study could have been sponsored by a vitamin manufacturer whose business was suffering, because they didn't put vitamin C in their products, and they were competing with other companies that did add vitamin C. Perhaps the research was done on a small group of people in nursing homes, who were about to die. This is a very extreme example illustrating how a study could be biased. Nonetheless, it is something you have to watch out for.

In general, the more studies have similar results, the more reliable the information is. You should be aware that a study is always conducted by a particular agency for a particular purpose and this can bias the results. As illustrated above, statistics cannot just be taken at face value. You have to interpret them. And you have to look at how the study interprets them, and what conclusions they draw from what statistics. For example, if a drug company is funding a study to test the effectiveness of a drug it is manufacturing, the company will want the results to be high: They want to show that their drug is effective so that they can sell it. This doesn't mean that the results are necessarily skewed or biased. It just means that it's important to learn who's conducting the study and what interests they have are in getting certain results.

Web resources

Hep-C-Alert
www.hep-c-alert.org/

Pubmed
www.pubmedcentral.nih.gov/
(The National Library of Medicine offers a free database. You can search a topic, and the database will provide summaries of scientific articles on your topic.):

American Association for the Study of Liver Diseases
www.aasld.org

Hep C Advocate
HCVadvocate.org

HepNet
www.hepnet.com
The Hepatitis Information Network is a source for both doctors and patients about viral hepatitis

Medline
www.nlm.NIH.gov/medline
US National Library of Medicine (NLM). The world's largest database of medical literature

Medscape
www.medscape.com

learning

Severe Liver Disease: Stages and Symptoms

IF YOU haven't experienced symptoms of severe liver disease, you may be wondering what they are. If you're like us, you may get scared reading about these symptoms. But remember that most people with hep C don't develop them. According to the CDC, people with hep C have:

○ A 10 to 20 percent chance of cirrhosis, usually over a period of 20 to 30 years
○ A 1 to 5 percent chance of mortality from chronic liver disease.

If you don't have severe liver damage now, and if you stay healthy, you have a good chance of never developing cirrhosis or any of the complications that we discuss below. Nonetheless it's important to know what they are.

What hepatitis C can do to the liver

The HCV virus primarily accumulates in the liver. Scientists believe it damages the liver in two ways—by invading liver cells and by triggering an immune response that destroys the cells. Chronic hepatitis, or chronic inflammation of the liver, can hinder the circulation of blood through the liver and cause liver cells to die. These dead cells harden, forming scar tissue on the liver. This buildup of fibrous scar tissue is called **fibrosis**. Although the liver can function efficiently even when large areas are scarred, the accumulation of fibrous tissue eventually impairs the circulation of blood through the liver and kills more cells. This means that the liver becomes less capable and efficient at storing nutrients and detoxifying the body's waste products and chemicals from outside.

The next stage of disease progression is **cirrhosis**, which means "scarring." Cirrhosis is the eighth leading cause of death in the United States. Out of 100 people with hep C, 10 to 20 will develop cirrhosis. Between one and four will develop liver cancer. In a cirrhotic liver, the accumulation of scar tissue is so severe that it impairs liver function and distorts the organ's structure and appearance. A cirrhotic liver looks bumpy instead of smooth, because nodules form on the surface, as the liver regenerates new cells. Cirrhosis prevents blood and lymph from flowing freely through the liver. Conventional western medicine has a hard time treating cirrhosis. Interferon is hard on a severely damaged liver. Thus many patients with cirrhosis are not eligible for interferon therapy, especially if they present the symptoms of **ascites** or **bleeding varices**, which we discuss below.

Cirrhosis may present no symptoms at all, in which case it is called "compensated cirrhosis." According to some studies, 50 percent of people with cirrhosis present no symptoms of end-stage liver disease even 15 years after they are first diagnosed. However, cirrhosis may also lead to some or all of the symptoms below.

Symptoms of cirrhosis

O Portal hypertension
O Bleeding varices
O Ascites

- ○ Edema
- ○ Encephalopathy
- ○ Coagulopathy
- ○ Jaundice
- ○ Pruritis
- ○ Weight loss
- ○ Osteoporosis

These symptoms can occur when the buildup of scar tissue prevents blood from flowing freely through the liver. This blood gets backed up in the **portal vein**—the vessel that collects blood from organs in the abdomen, including the stomach and intestines, and transports this blood to the liver. If the portal vein is blocked, the blood can't carry nutrients from the intestines to the liver. As blood collects in the portal vein, pressure builds, causing the vein to swell. This exerts pressure on the surrounding organs and causes the heart to work harder. The general name for this condition is **portal hypertension**.

Portal hypertension can cause symptoms such as **bleeding varices, ascites,** and **encephalopathy**.

As the blood gets backed up in the portal vein, blood vessels in the esophagus and stomach can also swell. **Bleeding varices** may develop. "Varices" are swollen veins—like varicose veins, only they're inside the body. These swollen veins may begin leaking blood. Small oozes might produce black stools. Larger amounts of bleeding may result in vomiting blood. If the varice ruptures or bleeds excessively, the patient may go into shock. This is a medical emergency that may require blood transfusions, vitamin K, drugs to stabilize blood pressure, or surgical procedures to repair the vein or route blood away from the liver to decrease portal hypertension. Extreme cases may require a liver transplant.

Ascites is the fluid retention in the abdomen. The swelling of the portal vein can block the lymph channels and cause lymph to spill into the abdomen, causing **ascites**, swelling of the abdomen, and sometimes **edema**, swelling of the legs. Low albumin levels in the blood also allow fluid to leak into the abdomen. People with ascites should restrict the sodium (salt) in their diet and possibly use **diuretics** (water pills) to help the kidneys get rid of water and salt. Most physicians prescribe a diuretic called spironolactone for ascites.

"My legs started swelling. I had no idea what was wrong with me. It was so weird. My doctor cut down my salt intake, and I had to change my diet. Turns out I had edema. Even worse than the edema was that my liver was failing. I have never been so tired or scared in my life."

—PAUL B.

Ascites is a sign of severely advanced liver disease. Many patients with ascites have reached a stage where they may need a liver transplant to survive. When a patient's abdomen is severely distended, it may be necessary to have a doctor drain the fluid by a process called **paracentesis** and determine the cause of ascites. By comparing albumin levels in the ascites to those in the blood, the doctor can tell whether the ascites is caused by liver disease. If ascites is accompanied by fever and high white blood cell count, the patient may have **spontaneous bacterial peritonitis (SBP)**, a bacterial infection in the abdomen, requiring antibiotic treatment. Most patients with SBP have mild to severe pain, but a third may have no symptoms except perhaps a change in their mental state. Loss of appetite and nausea are common symptoms, and it's possible to have SBP without a tender abdomen or fever.

When blood does not flow through the liver, the blood does not get filtered and still contains toxins and waste products. These include ammonia, which the liver produces during protein metabolism. A healthy liver neutralizes ammonia, but when the liver is not functioning efficiently, the buildup of ammonia and other toxins may be the cause of **encephalopathy**. The features of encephalopathy include cognitive and personality changes and neurologic disorders. Mild encephalopathy is characterized by lethargy, disorientation, and tremor. Severe cases may lead to coma.

This is a scary but potentially reversible condition. Treatment consists of correcting any fluid or electrolyte disorders and preventing toxins from being formed from proteins in the intestine. Laxatives (lactolose) or antibiotics (neomycin or metronidazole) may be used to kill intestinal bacteria, which produce ammonia from protein in the intestine. People with encephalopathy should be on a low-protein diet.

Some patients develop **coagulopathy**, meaning disturbances in blood clotting. People with this condition may bruise extremely easily and bleed profusely with minor cuts. Coagulopathy most often results from the liver being unable to make certain clotting factors from vitamin K. Patients may receive vitamin K supplement tablets (phytonadione). If you're experiencing any of these symptoms, avoid substances that prevent clotting, or "thin" the blood:

- Aspirin, Ibuprofen, Advil
- Vitamin E
- Garlic
- Ginger
- Fish oils
- Fenugreek
- Ginko Biloba
- Feverfew
- Ginseng.

Slowed blood clotting can increase one's risk of **hemorrhagic stroke**. In this type of stroke, a blood vessel in the brain leaks blood into brain tissue, causing damage. The underlying cause is usually a malformed blood vessel or high blood pressure, but a patient with slowed blood clotting may bleed to death. For this reason among others, coagulopathy may boost you right to the top of the transplant list.

Many patients with severe liver disease also experience **jaundice**, a yellow-orange discoloration of the skin caused by bilirubin. **Bilirubin** is formed from the natural breakdown of red blood cells. It is excreted in **bile**, which is the "sludge" the liver excretes into the intestine. Bile, which usually passes from the liver to the intestines, gets blocked and overflows into the body and builds up in the skin. The pigment bilirubin makes the skin and eyes turn yellow and can cause intense itching (**jaundice pruritis**). There are no specific treatments for pruritis caused by jaundice, although cholestyramine, a drug used to bind bile, may be helpful.

"My gums bleed every time I brush my teeth. My toothbrush is soaked with blood. My nose is bleeding all the time. I found out my platelet count is low. Therefore my blood isn't coagulating properly. I'm really scared, and one of the worst things is that I have to worry more about infecting other

people—like I can't kiss anyone because my gums are bleeding all the time."

—CANDACE K.

"I'm swollen with ascites, and I've had to be drained three times. It sounds gross but I'm used to it now. I can even tell if the ascites is infected by what the fluid looks like."

—CHRISTOPHER P.

Liver cancer or hepatocellular carcinoma (HCC)

As we mentioned above, 10 to 20 percent of people with hep C progress to cirrhosis and 1 to 4 percent develop liver cancer. Although scientists don't really know how hepatitis C causes liver cancer, they do know that alcohol is a factor. Other factors that contribute to liver cancer are cirrhosis, coinfection with hepatitis B, heavy smoking, older age and male sex. Hep C may become the leading cause of liver cancer in the United States. It is already the number one cause in Japan. Cancer is the extensive production of abnormal cells that can't carry out the function that they are supposed to. They multiply unchecked and basically clog up whatever organ or system they are in. Eventually, the abnormal cells crowd out the healthy cells so that even the healthy cells can't do their job.

In primary liver cancer, abnormal liver cells replace functioning liver cells. They usually don't metastasize or spread outside the liver. Many people who develop primary liver cancer have a poor life expectancy. Having liver cancer can boost you to the top of the transplant list, because a liver transplant may be the only way to prolong life. We talk more about transplants in the Learning section of Month 9.

Other conditions related to hepatitis C

- O Cryoglobulinema
- O Kidney disease
- O Arthritis

○ Thyroid disease
○ Skin conditions
○ Neuropathy.

There are other conditions that might be related to hepatitis C, including autoimmune disorders and lymphoma. Many doctors believe that hep C is a systemic illness—that is, a disease that affects the whole system, not just the liver. Nonetheless, most hep C research focuses on the liver, because the virus primarily accumulates there, causing inflammation of the liver, and because most western medical doctors specialize in one particular organ or part of the body: Hepatologists focus on the liver, cardiologists on the heart, and dermatologists on the skin, for instance.

Cryoglobulinemia is an immune disturbance, caused by immunoglobin, a type of antibody that the body produces to combat HCV. In this condition, proteins may clump together in the blood and damage the skin, nervous system, kidneys, eyes, brain, and heart. When this clustering occurs in the part of the kidney that filters blood (the **glomerulus**), it may cause plugging, which can damage the membrane and sometimes lead to kidney failure. Cryoglobulinemia may also cause intense itching, which can be uncomfortable and difficult to live with.

Many people with HCV have elevated levels of rheumatoid factors in their blood. Though this laboratory finding is often associated with **rheumatoid arthritis**, a condition characterized by joint pain and swelling, the arthritis commonly seen in patients with hep C is not rheumatoid arthritis.

Since the liver plays a role in regulating thyroid hormones, people with hepatitis C run a higher risk of developing **hypothyroidism**, the reduced production of thyroid hormones, or **hyperthyroidism**, the increased production of thyroid hormones. Five to 20 percent of hep C patients experience some sort of thyroid problem—most often hypothyroidism. The symptoms of hyperthyroidism include insomnia, weight loss, intolerance to heat, heart palpitations, and tremors. The symptoms of hypothyroidism include weight gain, sluggishness, intolerance to cold, dry skin, and mental confusion. Both of these conditions are treatable with medication.

Several skin conditions are sometimes associated with hepatitis C:

○ Lichen planus—a raised, reddish-brown spot
○ Lichenoid dermatitis—flat, scaly red patches on the skin
○ Porphyria cutanea tarda—blisters on parts of the skin exposed to light
○ Psoriasis
○ Purpura—a skin condition seen in cryoglobulinemia.

Cirrhosis diet

Although we discussed diet in Day 6, people with cirrhosis have special dietary considerations. They need to restrict their iron and salt intake. They also need protein, but it's important not to get too much protein. If you have cirrhosis, you need to consult your doctor and a dietician, who can evaluate how much protein your liver can handle. High levels of iron can lead to liver damage and can interfere with interferon therapy. People with advanced fibrosis and cirrhosis also need to watch their fat intake. A damaged liver has difficulty processing and eliminating fats. This can lead to elevated cholesterol and triglyceride levels. Unprocessed fat may make your stool light and greasy. Here are some tips to reduce your fat consumption:

○ Eat no more than three 3-ounce servings of meat a day. If you are experiencing encephalopathy, which is due to high levels of ammonia in the blood, don't eat red meat, which increases these levels.
○ Eliminate dairy products or use only low-fat dairy products.
○ Eliminate trans-fats. These are the fats that are solid at room temperature such as margarine. You can replace with trans-fats with oils such as canola, olive, and grapeseed.
○ Restrict sodium levels to less than 2000 mg a day. This means you shouldn't add salt to food that you are cooking or eating. Many prepared foods are high in sodium so check the labels carefully. Decreasing sodium will reduce the risk of fluid retention and ascites.

IN A SENTENCE:

Ten to 20 percent of people with hep C develop cirrhosis, and 1 to 4 percent develop liver cancer.

Finding a Counselor

IN WEEK 3 we talked about building a support system, which can consist of friends and family and possibly a hep C support group in person or online. By now—Month 8—you may have found that you have some issues that are difficult to discuss with your family and friends, because they all know each other or because they're too emotionally invested in the issue. In this case you might want to seek the help of a counselor.

Many people join a spiritual or religious group for spiritual and social support. If you want this kind of support, you can find a group that's right for you, whether you are Jewish, Christian, Pagan, Buddhist, Muslim, Hindu, or any other spiritual persuasion.

In any of these groups, you are likely to find people who can counsel you. The advantage of seeing a counselor from your spiritual group is that this person may share your values, cultural background, or ideals.

> *"I started going to NA about five years ago. My biggest problem with NA was the idea that I had to believe in a Higher Power. I'd been an atheist all*

*my life. I thought God was for cowards and fools. But I had
to get clean, so I tried thinking of my NA group as my Higher
Power. Then I tried thinking of my unconscious as my
Higher Power. Finally I took a meditation class at the Zen
center. Now I'm a practicing Buddhist."*

—JENNIFER W.

*"When I found out I had hep C, I went through a huge
period of hating myself. And I didn't want to tell anyone,
so I was holding it all inside. I had never been to church,
but I figured that at this point I had nothing to lose.
I started going and even went to confession. It felt great.
It allowed me to open up and talk to people.
And everyone in my church group is wonderful.
I love going to church. I feel as if it saved my life."*

—PAUL G.

Another source of support is a mental health professional—in other
words, a psychiatrist, psychoanalyst, psychologist, therapist, or social
worker. If you want to see a mental health professional, it's wise to interview at least several. You can ask your doctor and friends for referrals. Your
friends may be able to recommend therapists they have seen and tell you
what these therapists are like from a client's point of view. Find someone
outside your social circle, because one of the benefits of having a therapist
is that you can talk about your friends and family in a neutral setting with
someone who doesn't know them personally. It can also be disruptive to
your therapy if you're constantly running into your therapist at cocktail parties or on the golf course.

Interviewing mental health professionals

The most important thing is to find someone you can talk to. Whether
therapy helps you may depend more on you and on the skill of the individual therapist than on the kind of therapy that he or she practices.
Nonetheless, if you're not familiar with some of the different schools and

approaches, it's a good idea to learn about them and consider what might work best for you.

Do you want a psychiatrist, psychotherapist, a psychoanalyst, or a licensed clinical social worker? These distinctions depend on the kind of degree the person has. Psychiatrists, for example, have M.D.s. As medical doctors, they can prescribe psychiatric drugs, such as antidepressants. However, the fact that psychiatrists have been to medical school does not necessarily mean they're the best people to talk to. Some psychiatrists only prescribe drugs and don't do much talk therapy. As you interview mental health professionals, consider whether or not you'd want to take psychiatric medications and ask the people you interview if they tend to recommend drugs. If you're certain that you don't want to take meds, you may want to find someone who is not a psychiatrist, or find a psychiatrist who is into talk therapy. Some people, who want both talk therapy and medication, go to a psychotherapist or L.C.S.W. for talk therapy and a psychiatrist for meds. In some cases, your primary physician will prescribe medications in consultation with your psychotherapist or L.C.S.W.

Does your insurance cover this therapist or psychiatrist?

If not, you may consider seeing an intern if you have financial limitations. Although interns have less experience, the fact that they are new to the profession may also mean that they're less jaded and truly care about doing a good job. Lisa and Cara have both had good experiences with interns. Lisa had about 10 years of therapy, and it began with interns. The first two years she changed therapists several times, but when she finally found someone she liked, she kept seeing her for six and a half years. She thinks her years in therapy helped a lot.

When you find someone you like, stick with the therapy

Therapy can be a long-term process. It usually stirs up a lot of issues that are hard to deal with. You may be tempted to stop therapy when these issues come up, but this is a good indicator that your therapy is working.

"I lie to my therapist. I like her as a friend so much that I'm afraid she will get mad at me and stop liking me. Sometimes I do Ecstasy but am afraid to tell her because I don't want her to think less of me."

—GINA G.

IN A SENTENCE:

> *A counselor or mental health professional may be helpful in times of stress.*

learning

Demographics of Hep C and Travel Tips

Ethnic demographics of HCV

The prevalence of hepatitis C varies for different ethnic groups. The American Liver Foundation (ALF) gives the following demographics for the United States:

- O 3.2 percent of African Americans
- O 2 percent of Latinos
- O 1.2 percent of Caucasians.

According to the NHANES study of noninstitutionalized U.S. civilians, conducted between 1988 and 1994, no gender, racial, or ethnic group was independently associated with a higher risk of HCV infection.[1] Nonetheless the rates of hepatitis C infection in African American men are alarmingly high: 10 percent of the 30-to-49 age group has HCV. This high incidence is probably related to the fact that African American men have high rates of poverty, military service, and incarceration—circumstances that increase one's risk of hep C.

Prevalence of HCV in different age groups

In 2001 in the United States, the 30-to-39 age group had a 5 percent incidence of HCV—the highest of any age group. Experts speculate that this high rate of infection is due to IV drug use.

The prevalence of hep C in various age groups differs widely depending on the country. In Egypt, for instance, HCV is most prevalent in people over 50, due to the widespread use of contaminated syringes for vaccines from 1960 to 1980: between 7 and 15 million Egyptians contracted HCV when health care workers reused unsterilized needles during a campaign to immunize the population against the parasite schistosomiasis. In 2001, the HCV infection rates in Egypt were 45 percent in the over-50 age group, 30 percent in ages 30 to 39, and 5 percent in age 9 and under.[2]

Risk factors for developing chronic hep C

Chronic hepatitis C is defined as the persistence of HCV RNA in the blood for more than six months. While hep C becomes chronic in 75 to 85 percent of the people infected, some people have a better chance of clearing the virus than others. The risk of developing chronic hep C depends on factors such as the age at time of infection, gender, ethnicity, and the appearance of jaundice during the acute infection.

Younger people, especially those who contract hep C before age 20, are more likely to clear the virus. The NHANES study estimated the rate of progression to chronic hep C as 30 percent in people below age 20 and 76 percent in people over age 20. In the Dionysos study from Italy, the chronicity rate was 56 percent for people between age 12 and 25, and 87 percent for those over 25.[3]

Women, especially younger women, may have a lower rate of chronic infection. Evidence for this comes from follow-up studies after a medical accident in which large numbers of pregnant women in Germany and Ireland received shots of Rh immune globulin contaminated with HCV (genotype 1b). Among 704 Irish women who tested positive for HCV antibodies, the chronicity rate was 55 percent. The 917 German women who had been exposed to HCV also had a 55 percent chronicity rate. But these similar results may have to do with the fact that all these women contracted hep C the same way. The NHANES study and the Dionysos study showed that men and women had similar rates of chronic hep C.[4]

Different racial and ethnic groups have different rates of chronic infection. African Americans develop chronic hep C more often than whites and Latinos. In the NHANES, African Americans had an 86 percent chronicity rate, while whites had 68 percent. In surveys among IV drug users in inner-city Baltimore, African American men had a 95 percent rate. This high rate of chronic infection may be partly related to the fact that everyone surveyed was an IV drug user, which means they may have been exposed to HCV multiple times. African Americans also have a lower rate of sustained response to interferon-ribavirin therapy and twice the risk of liver cancer compared to whites. Asians have a four-times-greater risk of HCC than whites. Scientists have not identified any genetic differences that explain why different racial and ethnic groups have different rates of chronic infection, response to treatment, and HCC.[5]

Individuals who develop jaundice or other symptoms during the acute phase of infection are also more likely to clear the virus. For instance, of the 917 German women who received HCV-contaminated Rh immune globulin, those who became jaundiced had a 43 percent chronicity rate, while 60 percent of those with no history of jaundice went on to develop chronic HCV. Jaundice and other symptoms indicate that the patient's immune system is mounting a response to HCV and thus has a better chance of eradicating the virus. Jaundice in particular may be a sign of a more robust immune Th1 lymphocyte and cytokine response. The strength of the immune response plays a major role in determining whether a person develops chronic hep C and liver fibrosis. HIV-positive patients, especially those with a CD4 count of less than 200, have higher rates of chronic infection.

In summary, most people infected develop chronic hep C, but chronicity rates are higher in patients who are:

- older than 25
- male
- asymptomatic during acute infection
- African American
- HIV positive
- immunosuppressed.[6]

Risk factors for developing cirrhosis

Roughly 10 to 20 percent of people with hep C go on to develop cirrhosis. The risk of cirrhosis depends on factors such as alcohol use, age at time of infection, gender, degree of inflammation and fibrosis, and coinfection with HIV or hep B.

Drinking alcohol may accelerate the progression of fibrosis in people with hep C. The 2002 United States National Institutes of Health (NIH) Consensus Statement showed that 30 grams of alcohol a day increased the risk of liver damage in men with hep C, and 20 grams/day increased the risk in women. More moderate drinking may also contribute to fibrosis. The evidence is conflicting, but no study has shown that alcohol is not harmful to people with hep C. See Day 2 for more information.

Patients who contracted HCV at a younger age have a slower rate of fibrosis. People who become infected before age 40 have a 2 to 8 percent chance of developing cirrhosis within 20 years. People who contract the virus after age 40 have a 20 percent chance of progressing to cirrhosis in 20 years.[7]

Women have a 5 percent chance of developing cirrhosis, while men seem to have a 20 to 30 percent chance.[8] In the study of German woman who received HCV-contaminated Rh immune globulin, only 4 percent had cirrhosis after 20 years. In the study of Irish women who received contaminated Rh immune globulin, only 2 percent had "definite or probable" cirrhosis after 17 years, and 2 of the 7 women with cirrhosis said they were heavy drinkers.

Coinfection with HIV or HBV also accelerates liver scarring.

In summary, patients have a higher risk of cirrhosis if they:

○ drink 30 grams of alcohol a day for men, 20 for women
○ contract hep C when they are over 40
○ are male
○ show severe inflammation or advanced fibrosis on a liver biopsy
○ are coinfected with HIV or HBV.[9]

Poverty

According to the NHANES study, the biggest risk factors for nininstitutionalized U.S. civilians aged 17 to 59 were illegal drug use and high-risk sexual behavior, followed by poverty and lack of education.

While there are many poor people who don't engage in risky behavior, people living in poverty are more likely to have access to drugs, live in crowded or unsanitary conditions, and be incarcerated at some point. Also, more and more people with no or low income are ending up homeless. The University of California at Los Angeles conducted a study of 884 homeless and impoverished adults. Twenty-two percent were infected with HCV, while 1.4 percent had HIV. Lifetime injection drug users had the highest percentage of positive HCV antibody tests. The prevalence of hepatitis C among the homeless is still unknown, but many believe it is escalating.

Unfortunately, for the homeless and for most of the world, treatment for hepatitis C is too expensive. The poor and the incarcerated, two groups with a high incidence of HCV infection, also have little or no access to health care. Forty-three million people in the United States are uninsured. The states have inadequate federal funding, so in order to deal with the costs of programs such as Medicaid, they simply limit eligibility.

Two scientists in the UK are currently working with the Indian government to develop a cheaper alternative to pegylated interferon. They have redesigned Roche's version so that the large sugar molecule, which makes the medication last longer in the blood, is on the inside instead of the outside. An Indian company called Shantha, which produced the world's first cost-effective hepatitis B vaccine, has agreed to make the new medicine, and the Indian government will subsidize the clinical trials.

These cheaper drugs, called ethical pharmaceuticals, are versions of effective medications that have been structurally modified so that they are not covered under the patent of a large pharmaceutical company. Ethical pharmaceuticals are different from generic medications, which are exact copies of existing ones. The new drugs must still undergo rigorous clinical trials and then be submitted to a drug licensing body. The companies that manufacture ethical pharmaceuticals have to prove that their drugs are truly innovative and not just replicas. If approved, the new drugs could be used in developing countries where cost prohibits the majority of people from getting treatment. Unfortunately it may be harder to make these drugs available in industrialized nations. The multinational pharmaceutical companies will file patent suits to prevent cheaper, improved versions of their drugs from being sold in the United States or Europe.[10]

I grew up in a low-income community. I found out I have hep C last year. I had never heard of that before. When I heard how many people in my community might have it I was shocked. Why had we never heard of this? Why do so many black men have this disease and nobody talks about it? We know about AIDS but now there is this whole new thing. They don't care if we live or die.

—KIMBERLY D.

The prison population

Approximately one-third of the general prison population is infected with hepatitis C. This is a huge number of people. According to the U.S. Department of Justice, at the end of 2005, nearly 2.2 million people were incarcerated—the equivalent of 1 in every 136 U.S. residents. There are more than 7 million men and women in the U.S. correctional system, including on probation and on parole—about 3 percent of the U.S. adult population, or 1 in every 33 adults.

According to the *Western Journal of Medicine*, 39.4 percent of male inmates are HCV-positive (49.1 percent of these are white), and 53.5 percent of women inmates are HCV-positive, with the highest rate, 69.7 percent, among Latinas. A nonprofit group for prisoners with hepatitis C, the *Hepatitis C Awareness News*, states that incarcerated people represent one of the largest populations infected with hepatitis C.

Sixty-five percent of HCV-positive prisoners admitted to intravenous drug use. Of those with no history of drug use, inmates who had been incarcerated longer had higher rates of hep C. The CDC and American Public Health Association have issued guidelines to screen and manage hepatitis C in the prison system. Consequently, more prisons are testing inmates for hepatitis C, although many are only testing high-risk groups. And unfortunately, many prisons do not have the resources to comply with the CDC guidelines. If they test all the prisoners, then they may have to treat all of them, and some therapies run $10,000 to $20,000 per treatment. Voluntary clinical trials in prisons could provide much-needed research for both the inmate population and the population at large. This would have a national impact on the epidemic. But valid concerns that prisoners may be forced to participate or not be properly informed about new drugs have prevented clinical trials from happening in U.S. prisons.

The prison problem affects everyone. The number of state and federal releasees continues to increase each year. These are people who return to their communities and may continue to spread the virus, and, as their condition worsens, the community will have to bear the expense.[11]

> *People are shooting up in prison, and there is no way to get clean needles, forget about bleach. You can't even get condoms. People steal bread bags from the kitchen to use as condoms, if they even bother to do that much. It's no wonder that hep C is rampant.*
>
> —KEVIN K.

> *When I was locked up, it seemed like everyone had hep C. There were guys trying to get the Department of Corrections medical staff to approve interferon for them. A lot of people were very sick and weren't getting any treatment. The Department of Corrections has a huge problem with infectious diseases. I was in the California Correctional Center at Susanville. It's a fire camp training facility. The way it works is that the inmates have to pass a physical test before they go to the Department of Forestry to learn how to fight fire. And I was an inmate instructor who put them through the physical test. A lot of them were too sick to pass the test. And they don't do any medical treatment at the fire camp. The system is not treating them. It's warehousing them well, but it's not treating them for anything. The strongest thing you could get was Motrin.*
>
> —BRIAN S.

Veterans and hepatitis C

United States veterans have an unusually high rate of HCV infection. Vietnam-era veterans have the highest incidence of HCV, followed by

Korean War vets, World War II vets, and Persian Gulf vets. According to the *VA Cooperative Study 488* (2005)—the largest study of veterans to date—5.4 percent of veterans enrolled in VA health care are infected with hep C. This is lower than previous studies (ranging from 6.6 percent to 35 percent), but higher than the rate of infection in the general population (1.8 percent).

The actual number of veterans infected with hep C is unknown, because studies have only included veterans using the VA health care system, an estimated 17 percent of the almost 27 million U.S. veterans. Many veterans are homeless or use other health care systems.

The *VA Cooperative Study 488* claims that military service had no impact on spreading hepatitis C and that the two-fold increase of HCV infection in veterans is due to increased exposure to traditional risk factors. The rate of hepatitis C is higher among vets who have used IV drugs, have tattoos, and those who have spent more than 48 hours in prison. No study has found that active-military personnel have a higher rate of HCV than the general population.

Nonetheless, many veterans believe that active duty in the military put them at higher risk. HCVets.com states that before 1996, no standard precautions for medical personnel were in place. It was common practice to reuse devices such as high-speed jet injectors (airguns), needles, and vials that held multidose vaccines. Medical personnel also used stainless steel and glass syringes—neither of which could be properly sterilized. Finally, the same strain of HCV has been found in people who were vaccinated in the same unit, at the same time, with the same gun. HCVets.com claims that the *VA Cooperative Study 488* concentrated too heavily on multiple sex partners as a risk and not enough on exposure to vaccinations by high-speed jet guns.

Hepatitis C accounts for 55 percent of all liver transplants at the VA, and there are over 200,000 veterans in treatment. This is a huge burden on the VA system. At the same time, many veterans are not candidates for treatment due to psychiatric disorders or drug or alcohol abuse. Moreover, many veterans are not getting tested because they do not think they fit into the high-risk categories, such as drug abuse or multiple sex partners, designated by the Veteran Affairs Department. It is important for every veteran to get tested. The numbers of infected veterans may be higher than VA estimates due to many possible risk factors:

○ Short supply of medical equipment; reused needles, vials, or connectors
○ Vaccine contaminations, high-speed jet injections
○ Exposure to blood during combat and combat training
○ Medical care under unsanitary conditions
○ Transfusions before blood was screened in 1992
○ Service in areas with high rate of infection, including Asia and North Africa
○ High rate of drug use
○ Crowded living conditions; sharing toiletries such as razors.

For more information visit the Web site for veterans with hep C at http://www.hcvets.com. This site also has a bulletin board.[12]

Foreign travel

No matter where you are, it's best to take standard precautions and avoid exposure to blood. International travelers should avoid medical, dental, and cosmetic procedures, blood transfusions in countries where the blood supply might not be screened for HCV, acupuncture, IV drugs, and tattooing under nonsterile conditions. IV drug use is the most commonly reported way U.S. citizens contract HCV abroad, followed by transfusions and other medical procedures involving blood products. If you drive in a foreign country, don't drive too fast or while intoxicated, because car accidents are the main reason international travelers need transfusions.

Some countries have higher hepatitis C rates than others: in parts of Africa, Asia, and South America, the incidence of HCV exceeds 10 percent. As we discussed in Day 1, different genotypes are more prevalent in different continents. It is possible to contract more than one strain of HCV, which may result in a more virulent infection. This may sound scary, but if you are careful, the risk of contracting hep C while traveling is low.

If something goes wrong, the safest thing to do is contact your embassy or one of the international travelers' assistance organizations listed below. Write down any allergies or illnesses and the names of emergency contacts, and keep this information in your passport. If you are on medication, carry the medication on your person or in your carry-on luggage. It's not always easy or safe to get prescriptions filled in a foreign country, so carry an extra up-to-date, legible prescription or statement from your doctor including the medication's trade name, manufacturer, chemical name, and dosage.

The Immunization Action Coalition recommends that everyone with hepatitis C get vaccinated for hepatitis A, hepatitis B, influenza, pneumo-coccal disease, tetanus, and diphtheria before traveling anywhere. Contracting any of these illnesses on top of hepatitis C can hurt your liver, and coinfection with HAV or HBV can be deadly. Make sure to check if the country you are visiting requires any additional vaccines. If you want to work abroad, some countries require entrance tests for hepatitis B, hepa-titis C, and HIV. Countries such as Kuwait and Malaysia may deny you a visa for a positive test. You can check the U.S. State Department for vac-cine and visa information. The World Health Organization urges anyone doing humanitarian relief work abroad to be careful of exposure to blood or any bodily fluids in health care settings.

Tips for traveling

O Learn something about the conditions and medical practices in the countries you are visiting.

O When you are visiting a country where the blood supply might not be screened for HCV, or medical equipment may not be sterilized, make sure you know where the best facilities are and where they perform medical procedures under sterile conditions. You can always call your embassy for recommendations.

O Get all the recommended vaccinations for the country in which you are traveling. Find out if there are any additional diseases that you may be exposed to in those areas. If there are vaccines for these diseases, get them as well.

O Even if the particular country you're visiting does not require HAV and HBV vaccines, make sure you get them before you travel. This may mean waiting six months, but it is very important. Contracting HAV or HBV on top of hep C could be fatal.

O Try to avoid any invasive medical procedures, including shots, IVs, transfusions, and cosmetic procedures.

O Think twice before getting acupuncture, a tattoo, or a piercing in another country. In the United States, acupuncture, tattoo, and piercing parlors have to meet regulations. Everything is sterilized using regulated equipment such as autoclaves. This may not be the case elsewhere.[13]

For more information on travel precautions, call one of these organizations.

U.S. Department of State
202-647-5225
travel.state.gov
CDC International Traveler's Health Information Line: 877-394-8747
www.cdc.gov/travel

Healthcare Abroad
243 Church Street West
Vienna, VA 22180
800-237-6615

International Association for Medical Assistance to Travelers
417 Center Street
Lewiston, NY 14902
716-754-4883
IAMAT
1623 Military Rd. #279
Niagara Falls, NY 14304-1745
716 754 4883
www.iamat.org/

International SOS Assistance
P.O. Box 11568
Philadelphia, PA 19116
800-523-8930
www.internationalsos.com

MONTH 9

living

Networking with Others: Get Involved!

"In ten years we will have as many liver benefits as we now do for breast cancer."

—LINDA C.

MANY OF us had never heard of hepatitis C until we were diagnosed with it. With 300 million people infected worldwide, it's shocking that we aren't more informed. Hepatitis C is a global epidemic, which will kill more people than HIV. Yet most political leaders are in denial about it. We need to raise public awareness of this epidemic globally as well as locally. One way to learn about hepatitis C and become more proactive in your health care is to teach others about HCV.

Getting involved may help you emotionally as well. Even with 300 million infected with HCV, the lack of media attention can leave us feeling alone. Getting involved in an HCV community in your area or on-line may help you feel less isolated.

Another reason to get involved is because our government doesn't fund hepatitis C research nearly enough. We may feel powerless because there are no effective treatments, and it may seem as if research isn't moving fast enough to help us.

Activism can make a difference and allow us to feel as if we're doing something.

To figure out what type of community involvement you might like, you may want to consider whether you are interested in support, political activism, or both.

Get involved in support groups

As we said in Week 3, your family and friends may not understand everything you're going through. Other people with hep C can often validate your emotional issues and any symptoms you're experiencing. They can share their experiences on the latest treatments and ways of dealing with the day-to-day hardships of living with hep C. If you're considering interferon, it is especially helpful to talk to other people who are undergoing the same treatment. They may be able to suggest ways to mitigate some of the side effects.

You can find local support groups by calling your local hospital, or a national liver or hepatitis foundation. There are many resources for support groups, and lots of them are online.

Priority Healthcare Corporation
www.hepatitisneighborhood.com

Hepatitis A, B, and C Prevention Programs
Lists many different support groups.
www.hepprograms.org/support/hepc.asp

Hepatitis-central.com
hepatitis-central.com/hcv/support/main.html (Lists worldwide support groups as well.)

HepCPrimer.com
www.hepcprimer.com/patient/support.html

Objective Medicine
www.objectivemedicine.com (See section on support groups.)

If you are interested in political activism

○ Volunteer at a liver or hepatitis organization.
○ Write letters to your local congressional representative.
○ Participate in liver walks.
○ Organize benefits.

○ Lobby.
○ Donate. Be sure that you choose an organization that donates most of its money to research and treatment.

The Web site HepatitisActivist.org has e-mail petitions you can automatically send to your local politicians. The American Liver Foundation (www.liverfoundation.org) also has petitions in circulation and up-to-date information.

> *"I've gotten really into writing letters to my congressman. I go to this Web site with prewritten letters. I have sent many of my friends there. It's heartwarming to know that even my friends who don't have hep C are willing to help."*
>
> —TONY R.

IN A SENTENCE:

> *Getting involved may help you feel less isolated and more proactive about your healthcare.*

learning

Become an Organ Donor: Liver Transplants Save Lives!

"A liver transplant is truly the gift of life. I would be dead if that organ donor and her relatives had not donated her liver to me."

—LYNN T.

HEPATITIS C now ranks as the number one cause of fatal liver disease: 10 percent of people with hepatitis C progress to end stage cirrhosis and 5 percent of those with cirrhosis develop liver cancer. Presently, the only treatment for end-stage liver disease is **liver transplant surgery**—the process of removing a liver that no longer functions and replacing it with a healthier liver taken from the body of an organ donor. This is one of the most radical procedures of modern medicine. Called the "gift of life," transplantation is a last resort procedure—performed only on people who would die without a new liver. Many transplant recipients have waited on the transplant list for years. Many of these people have also lived for years with debilitating liver disease, and the new organ restores their health and vitality, along with all the vital functions that the liver performs.

People who receive transplants have an 80 percent chance of surviving five years. The survival rate may be lower for transplant recipients who had HCC. Unfortunately, transplants are not a cure for hep C. The virus almost always infects the new liver, and frequently the disease progresses much faster in transplant recipients, who have to take immunosuppressive drugs to prevent their bodies from rejecting the new organ. Transplant recipients thus have a 25 percent chance of cirrhosis in the next five years. This is much higher than the rate in the general hep C population. Scientists are researching treatments for HCV-positive transplant recipients. The combination of **interferon** and **ribavirin** looks promising.[1]

Another problem is the lack of organ donors. Since the first transplant in 1963, surgeons have performed more than 81,000 liver transplants in the United States alone. Nonetheless, the demand for new livers far outweighs the supply. Each year approximately 6,000 people receive liver transplants, but many die waiting for them. Without more organ donors, these numbers will skyrocket, as deaths from hepatitis C are expected to triple over the next 10 to 20 years. It is in our best interest to do everything in our power to promote organ donation.

The first thing we can do is become organ donors. Most states allow you to sign a form stating that you wish to be an organ donor. In some states, the signature or some other symbol appears on your driver's license. But many organ donor organizations will also contact your closest relatives and obtain their consent before they use your organs for transplants. Therefore, if you want to donate your organs, it's important that you express your wishes to your nearest of kin. Many people prefer to avoid these kinds of conversations, but it only takes a few words, and it may save someone's life. To make doubly sure, you can sign a witnessed or notarized agreement, clearly stating your intentions.

Transplant misconception #1: People with HCV cannot donate organs.

It's a common misconception that people with hep C cannot donate organs. However, many people with hep C have healthy, functioning livers for decades after infection. If you become an organ donor, your organs can save the life of someone else with hep C. Like blood products, donor organs are screened for HCV, HBV, and other antibodies. If an organ tests positive for HCV or HBV, it is called a **core-positive organ**, and it is offered to someone who has antibodies for HCV, HBV, or both. Thus, someone with HCV or HBV can receive a liver that is infected with HCV or HBV. Although it's possible for a HCV-positive transplant recipient to contract HBV or a different strain of HCV, the transplant will still prolong his or her life.

Misconception #2: Organ donation is a racket.

In the United States, the decision as to who receives a transplant is made by a team of doctors and social workers who consider many factors. It's an extremely careful evaluation process, and usually what it comes down to is who is most likely to survive.

Many people have heard urban legends about people waking up in their bathtubs with their kidneys missing, or they've heard that organs are stolen from the poor and given to the rich and famous. It's true that there's a thriving black market that pays third world people minuscule amounts of money for their kidneys, eyes, and other organs. A Johns Hopkins study also found some inequities in liver transplantation in the United States: According to this study, women, children, Latinos, and Asian-Americans wait longer for a transplant, and women, older patients, Asian-Americans, and African-Americans are more likely to die on the waiting list.[2] Occasionally celebrities receive transplants faster than people who are not famous. This celebrity privilege affects relatively few people, however. The scarcity of donor organs is a far greater problem.

Factors that can make you more eligible for a transplant

Today over 17,000 people are waiting for liver transplants in the United States. The wait list for liver transplants is incredibly long. Some people wait for over two years and others die waiting for them. The main factors affecting how soon you get a transplant include how quickly you will die without one and how likely you are to survive with a new organ. Having liver cancer or another immediately life-threatening illness can boost you to the top of the list. If you think that someday you might need a transplant, it's important to keep in mind that these factors may make you more eligible.

○ Leading an alcohol- and drug-free lifestyle. Some people think this is unfair. But it is less so when you consider the short supply of donor organs and the fact that alcohol and drugs are so damaging to the liver, that transplant recipients who drink and do drugs are much less likely to survive. The doctors who evaluate potential recipients don't want to give an organ to someone who's not going to take care of it.

○ Having a good support system. If you are getting a transplant you absolutely need people to help take care of you and follow the complicated medical regimen. You will need help with everything from buying your groceries to taking your medication. You will also need people to monitor you for danger signs. People with a good support system have a much higher rate of surviving.

○ Keeping up with your medical care. If you have severe liver damage, it's a good idea to get your name on the list as soon as possible. Being an active patient helps the transplant team know that you are serious about your recovery. Keeping all of your appointments and making extra effort is a show of good faith. If you have liver cancer, you must have regular scans to ensure that the cancer isn't spreading so much that you will no longer be eligible for a transplant.

○ Being mentally and emotionally stable. Transplants cause a lot of anxiety and sometimes depression. Some people see mental health professionals or seek spiritual or religious guidance. No matter how you do it, it's vital that you are emotionally stable.

○ Having health insurance. Transplants are very expensive, costing an average of $250,000. It's nearly impossible to get government programs such as Medicaid to pay for transplants, unless you are completely destitute. Moreover, the better health insurance you have, the better transplant facility you can go to, and the better care you will receive. If you have a low income, keep in mind that there are some areas of the country where Medicaid and other government programs provide more financial support for transplants and other medical needs. Ask your doctor to refer you to a social worker who can talk to you about your options.

In addition to making yourself more eligible for a transplant, there are things you can do to give yourself a better chance of surviving it. Choose a good transplant center. There are 117 transplant centers in the United States. Choose a surgeon who is very experienced in performing transplants and a center that has performed at least 20 transplants a year. This indicates that the center is efficient and effective at performing transplants. Ask about the survival rate of transplant recipients.

"I was on the transplant list and knew my name was coming up. I had no idea what time or what day they would call, so I got a cell phone. I could hardly sleep. I was at a friend's house when the doctor called me. I remember the time on my cell phone exactly. It was 3:41 in the afternoon on April 22, 1999. The doctor at the transplant unit said that they had a liver for me, I had to leave immediately. My friend drove me to the hospital."

—BARRY K.

"When I got my transplant, I got a 'core-positive' organ, which meant it tested positive for antibodies to hep C. It doesn't matter, because it was a healthy organ, and my hep C would have infected the new liver anyway. Infected or not, this liver saved my life. I think about how my donor may have known she had hepatitis C and donated her organ thinking it would save the life of someone else who had hep C just like her."

—JILL M.

"I just got my new liver. I'm so relieved because I was going to die. It's not over yet, though. It's possible that the virus could attack my new organ really aggressively and I could get cirrhosis really fast."

—ISABEL W.

Living donors: You don't have to be dead to donate!

The type of transplant that we have been talking about so far is a **cadaveric transplant**, in which the new organ comes from someone who has recently died. A more recent innovation is the **living donor liver transplant**: 40 to 60 percent of a living person's liver is removed and put into the body of someone who needs a liver. Since the liver can regenerate three-fourths of its tissue in a few weeks, both the donor and recipient have fully functioning livers a few months after the operation. As of 2006, almost 78,000 cadaveric transplants and more than 3,000 living-donor transplants had been performed in the United States.

Since the late 1980s surgeons have been doing parent to child liver transplants. In the early 90s they began doing adult to adult live donor transplants. Often the donors are family members. They need to have a compatible blood type, but unlike in other transplants, the tissue type doesn't have to be compatible.

While some doctors and scientists view this as a possible solution to the shortage of organs, others maintain that not enough study has been done. There are in fact ethical considerations. Most living donors are partners or family members of the potential transplant recipient, who is going to die because no other livers are available. One ethical consideration is that some living donors may not be taking their own safety into account because they are so concerned about saving their loved one. Since living donors are carefully screened, death and other complications are rare. The death rate is 0.5 to 1 percent. About one-third of living donors are rejected due to a medical condition that could endanger their health or life. Still, some people suggest that a government agency should regulate the process of selecting living donors and monitoring their safety.

> *"After my transplant, they put me on steroids.*
> *The steroids gave me so much energy that*
> *people had to force me to sit down."*
>
> —LILLIAN K.

Split-liver transplants

In a split-liver transplant, the liver of a deceased donor is divided into adult and child-size portions. The larger part goes to an adult, and the smaller part goes to a child. In the past, many children with end-stage liver disease died waiting for transplants. As split-liver transplants become more common for young children, they will reduce the mortality rate of kids on the waiting list.

Check-in

○ Have you gotten your second round of hepatitis A and B vaccines?

○ Have you gotten your liver panels recently? It's a good idea to get them every three months for the first two years. After you receive your diagnosis. By Month 9, you should have had two or three liver panels, and hopefully you're keeping your test results on file with your medical records. If you haven't gotten a liver panel recently, schedule one. Then compare the results of your last three or four panels.

○ Become an organ donor. In some states, your nearest kin will have the last word, so you may need to discuss this with them. It isn't a topic people generally like to discuss, but it only takes a few minutes to tell them that you want to be an organ donor.

○ If you haven't already gotten a liver biopsy, talk to your doctor about scheduling one.

IN A SENTENCE:

> *You can still be an organ donor, even if you have hep C: Liver transplants save lives!*

living

Children and Hep C

WHETHER TO have children is one of the major decisions you will make or have made in your lifetime. Having hepatitis C makes this decision even harder. Children are a huge responsibility even if a patient does not have a chronic illness. Those of us who want children may fear that we will transmit the virus to our kids or get too sick to care for them. Some of us also worry that potential partners may shy away from us if they want to have kids.

> *I met the greatest girl. We were having a*
> *wonderful relationship, but as it grew more*
> *serious, she grew more distant. After weeks of*
> *asking her, she finally admitted to me that she*
> *really wanted to have kids, but she wasn't sure if*
> *she wanted the father of her children to have a*
> *chronic illness. I was devastated.*
>
> —SAM T.

Can I transmit hep C during pregnancy or birth?

Vertical transmission refers to transmission of the virus from mother to child, usually during birth. According to the

CDC, the risk of perinatal transmission is 4 percent for mothers who have hep C but are not coinfected with HIV. This low risk can still make the decision to have children very frightening. A caesarian section is not recommended, though the risk seems the same whether the baby is born vaginally or by caesarian. The risk of vertical transmission jumps to 19 percent when the mother is coinfected with HIV and HCV. Perinatal transmission rates may be higher in nonindustrialized countries, due to nonsterile conditions.

While the fetus is in the uterus, it usually tests positive for HCV antibodies. Through a process called **passive transfer,** antibodies to hep C cross the mother's placental barrier and become detectable in the fetus's blood. These antibodies usually remain detectable for a period of three to six months after birth. They do not indicate whether the child is infected with hep C. Unfortunately they don't prevent the child from contracting hep C either. If the antibodies are still detectable after one year, the baby is diagnosed with chronic hepatitis C.

It is unlikely that breastfeeding increases the risk of hep C. The risk may be higher if the mother is experiencing symptoms of hep C, or if she has cracked or broken skin on her nipples.

If you already have kids

> *My mommy has hep C. She told me what it is and told me how important it is that I don't touch blood. I love my mommy, and I'm scared when she gets sick.*
>
> —PATRICK A.

What if you already have kids when you're diagnosed with hep C? As we emphasize in Day 2, the first things you can do are:

O Take **standard precautions**, the CDC's guidelines for preventing the transmission of blood-borne pathogens (like hep C, HIV, and hep B). As we discussed in Day 2 Learning, these precautions involve wearing latex or polyurethane gloves when you come into contact with any body fluid except sweat, unless you can easily contain the fluid with a thick cloth or nonporous material. Teach your children standard precautions (see guidelines below for teaching children ages 2 to 7), and make sure your child's school or day care center practices standard precautions.

O Get your kids tested for hep C.

O Tell your children how hep C is transmitted, if they are old enough to understand. In the next section, we discuss how to talk to kids of different ages.

O Put away razors, toothbrushes, hairbrushes, nail clippers, and other personal items that may be contaminated with your blood. This is especially important if your children are too young to understand how hep C is transmitted.

O Some kids like to poke themselves and play with sharp objects like needles in a sewing kit. It's also popular for adolescents to pierce their ears. Explain to your kids why this is dangerous and discourage them from doing this at home with their friends. You may want to take them to a professional to get their ears (or any other body part) pierced.

Children with hep C

There are several ways children can contract hep C.

O Before 1992 many adolescents with conditions such as hemophilia, leukemia, thalessemia, and congenital heart disease got hep C through blood transfusions and blood products.

O Some children acquire HCV **perinatally**—that is, from their mothers during birth.

O Some children and adolescents contract the virus by sharing works used for IV drugs.

O Some children and adolescents get it through household risks or through sexual activity, though these are rarely modes of transmission.

No matter how a child contracts hep C, the diagnosis is often devastating for both the child and the parents or caretakers.

If your child has hep C: Deciding whom to tell

My child and I both have hep C. I am worried about telling his teacher because I don't want him to be treated

*differently. I know that he can't be pulled out of school, but
I am more concerned about his self-esteem. I am especially
worried about other children finding out and teasing him or
avoiding him.*

—HELEN F.

When parents learn that their child has hep C, their first impulse is
often to talk about the diagnosis with family and friends, but it is important to exercise great care in deciding whom to tell. Once you share information with someone, you can never take it back. Telling one person is
often tantamount to telling everyone, and it's not uncommon for a child
with hep C to be excluded from family events, community activities, and
even day care or school.

If you have just learned your child has hep C, it is wise not to share this
traumatic news with anyone except immediate family and health professionals until you are feeling less distraught and can make informed choices
about whom to tell.

Here are some questions to ask yourself before you tell someone:

○ Does this person need to know? Do they provide child care? Would
it be sufficient to make sure this person is taking standard precautions rather than disclosing your child's HCV status?
○ Is this person generally compassionate towards others? Have they
been supportive toward you in the past?
○ How much do they know about infectious diseases?
○ Have you heard them make comments about people with HIV or
hep C? Are they sympathetic? Fearful?
○ Have they been able to keep confidences in the past, or are they
likely to tell others?

Health professionals

Parents are not obligated to disclose their child's hep C status to doctors,
nurses, dentists, or other health care workers, but it is generally safe to do
so. It is illegal for health professionals to share information about a patient's
medical conditions without the patient's or guardian's consent. It may not

matter whether you tell your child's dentist before a routine teeth cleaning, but telling your child's pediatrician is important even if your child is being treated for other conditions. Health care workers can make more informed medical decisions if they know the child has hep C.

Schools, daycare centers and camps

It is not necessary to disclose a child's HCV status to a school, day care center, or camp, because the staff should be handling first-aid situations according to **standard precautions**, the CDC's guidelines for preventing the transmission of blood-borne pathogens (like hep C, HIV, and hep B). As we discussed in Day 2 Learning, these precautions involve wearing latex or polyurethane gloves when you come into contact with any body fluid except sweat, unless you can easily contain the fluid with a thick cloth or nonporous material. Since the basic principle is to assume that everyone's blood and body fluids contains pathogens, it's not necessary to single out individuals with infectious diseases and treat them differently. As we mentioned, 40 to 90 percent of people with infectious diseases don't know they have them. As the American Academy of Pediatrics *Red Book* states, "routine use of these precautions avoids the necessity of identifying children known to be infected with HIV, HBV, and HCV and acknowledges that unrecognized infection poses at least as much risk as the identified child."[1]

It is generally a good idea for parents to make sure that a school or day care center standard precautions before enrolling their children. In some cases, parents of children with hep C have sent the school an anonymous letter stating that one of the students had hep C and enclosing information about standard precautions. This is a good compromise because it protects the child's privacy while ensuring that the school is informed.

Sports events

The American Academy of Pediatrics *Red Book* states, "Because of the low probability of transmission of their infection to other athletes, athletes infected with HIV, hepatitis B, or hepatitis C should be allowed to play sports."[2] If the coaches are taking standard precautions, parents can feel safe.

Babysitters, play dates and sleepovers

These are gray areas, because you can't assume that babysitters and other parents are trained in standard precautions. The American Red Cross recommends that parents provide latex or polyurethane gloves for babysitters to use when handling blood and other body fluids.

It's hard to know how to handle play dates and sleepovers. Each family has to make its own decision. Once the child old enough to know how to handle his or her own blood spills, it probably isn't necessary to inform anyone. Parents of small children may want to inform the other parents if they know them well.

PKIDs provides the following guidelines for how to share information about a child's hep C diagnosis:

○ Determine who needs to know.
○ Find out what they know about hep C.
○ Try to guess their possible reactions, and prepare yourself mentally.
○ Tell them about the diagnosis (and ask them not to mention it to the child or to anyone else).
○ Give them some educational material on hep C and standard precautions so they will know what to do.[3]

My children all know not to use each other's toothbrushes. But my hep C positive daughter had a friend spend the night, and her friend used her toothbrush. Now I have to tell the girl's parents, and I don't know how I'm going to do that.

—WENDY B.

IN A SENTENCE:

Teach your children standard precautions and think carefully before telling anyone about your child's hep C.

learning

Teaching Kids About Hep C

Talking to children ages 2 to 7

It is best not to tell young children about hepatitis C, because they probably won't understand the disease or its ramifications. Before age five, kids have a hard time telling the difference between real and imaginary threats. They also tend to repeat things they hear. If you tell a small child he has have hep C or that someone in the family has hep C, he will probably spread the news. Adults frequently make mistakes about whom they tell about an infectious, stigmatized disease, but a young child lacks the knowledge and communication skills to educate people about hep C, as well as the ability to discern who is safe to tell and who may treat him badly. Needless to say, this could create additional troubles for the family.

While small children may not be able to understand hep C, no child is too young to learn basic standard precautions. PKIDs offers suggestions for role-playing standard precautions with children:

○ Teach your child how invisible germs spread from one person to another by putting glitter on her hands and letting her play with family members, go to the bathroom, and touch a cracker without eating it. Then take her back to the beginning of the glitter trail and follow it—illustrating how germs spread. Show her how to prevent the spread of germs by washing off the glitter.

○ Teach your child not to touch another person's blood. Have someone "bleed" ketchup. Have your child to run and get a grown-up when she sees blood. Then pretend that no grown-ups are around, and show her how to use a plastic bag or towel to clean up the blood without touching it with her bare hands.

○ If your child does not understand why she shouldn't touch other people's blood or let others touch hers, ask her if she would touch someone else's poop or snot. When you get a resounding "no," explain that blood is another personal thing they shouldn't touch.[4]

When children reach the age of five or six, you can explain why these precautions are necessary. As suggested above, keep razors, nail clippers, and other items that can break skin where your children can't get them. If you have more than one child, you may want to write each of your children's names on their toothbrushes. You can use a glittery nontoxic paint and make it a fun art project and make sure they understand that this is one thing they should not share.

Here are some more things parents of young children can do:

○ Communicate with your child about visits to doctors and hospitals, shots, blood draws, etc. Be ready to help her through procedures that may be frightening and painful. Depending on the child's age and attention span, you may be able to teach her some breathing techniques to deal with fear and anxiety.

○ Decide whom to tell (See suggestions in the "Whom to Tell" section.)

○ Be ready to advocate for your child at school or day care.

○ Be conscious of how your body language transmits info to your child before you tell him about hep. If you send out "fear rays" when you enter a doctor's office, your child will pick up on this and become anxious.

○ Even if you can't talk about hep, you can speak generally of why they are seeing the doctor and what to expect. Assure your child that the doctor's appointment or blood draw is not a punishment for something she's done.

If your child asks why she has to see the doctor all the time when other kids don't, point out that everyone is unique. Another kid wears glasses, another has red hair, etc. If she asks why she has to go to the doctor again or have her blood drawn again, explain that sometimes things change, and the doctor has to know about the changes.

Your kid may have to answer questions about why he has so many medical appointments, or why he is missing so much school. Teach him to answer politely with general information, such as "I was sick, but now I'm better." Practice with your child so he knows how to respond to these queries.

If your child is afraid of trips to the doctor's office or hospital:

○ Tell her when and where she's going several days in advance.
○ Don't promise that this visit will be easier than past visits, because this may not be true, and your child needs to be able to trust you.
○ Pack a travel bag with a favorite toy or reassuring photo.
○ Show your child that you are fixing up her room for her return. This will assure her that she'll be back soon.
○ If your child has frequent doctor's appointments, hang a calendar on her wall and put a sticker on every date that she goes to the doctor without complaining.

Deal with fear of pain by asking the child what she imagines will happen. Assure her that the doctor will do everything in his power not to cause too much pain. Accept that she will respond to pain with tears, confusion, and anger. These are normal responses. Don't punish her for them. Respond with love, comfort, and support.

If a parent is very sick due to complications of cirrhosis, it is futile to hide this from a child. Break it to the child slowly, building on what she already knows about disease and her parent's illness. Most children are aware of the finality of death by the time they reach age six to ten. You may want to enlist a counselor or therapist to help a child come to terms with a parent's life-threatening illness and possible death.

Children 8 to 12

By this time, the child has more understanding of cause and effect. She understands that people can die from a disease, injury, or accident. She is less likely to fear monsters and other imaginary creatures and more likely to fear real people who might hurt her. Being honest with her will show her that you respect her intelligence and tell her about important things.

Lori W. Wiener, the coordinator of the Pediatric HIV Psycho-Social Support and Research Program at the National Institutes of Health, and Heidi Haiken, the coordinator of Social Work at the Francois Xavier Bagnoud Center in Newark, New Jersey, have spent many years helping parents talk with their children about their HIV status. The PKIDs Pediatric Hepatitis Report cites Wiener and Haiken's two cardinal rules for disclosing to kids:

Never lie. You don't have to tell young children the name of the disease, but don't lie. Your child needs to trust you, and lying will only damage your relationship. Educate your child about hep C gradually—building on what she already knows. "Remember how I said there was a germ in your blood? That germ is a virus named hepatitis C." If the child asks, "Why didn't you tell me earlier," you have to be able to say, "I never lied to you. I told you what was the matter, I just didn't tell you that the virus was called hepatitis C."

Tell the child as soon as you can—as soon as he begins asking questions. Don't wait until your child is 12 to tell him about a disease he's had for years that you've never mentioned. Disclosing gets harder the longer you wait, and you run the risk of losing your child's trust. He may feel upset or embarrassed that other family members knew about his diagnosis before he did. Usually everyone feels better after the disclosure. The parents and older siblings are relieved, and the child, who probably intuited that something was up, feels better now that he knows. He may take months or years to absorb the information about hep C. Encourage him to share his feelings and ask questions no matter how hard it is to talk about.[5]

Disclosing can be devastating for the parents, even if they had nothing to do with the child contracting hep C. Parents who used IV drugs in the past and infected their child may feel excruciating guilt that their son or daughter has to suffer. Some parents may need to resolve their own issues around guilt and their past before they disclose. It's important that the parents or caregivers, rather than a doctor, tell the child.

○ Some parents find it helpful to write out how they will tell their child about hep C and then have a family member or counselor role-play the part of the child. As you decide what to tell your child, keep in mind the most important message you want to convey. This might be: "I will always be there for you," "I will never lie to you," or "You don't have this disease because you did something wrong."

○ Build on what your child already knows or what you have already told him about infections: "Remember when you had that blood draw?" or "Remember when I told you not to touch someone else's blood?"

○ Be prepared to answer the following questions, depending on your child's age and whether you or your child is infected.
  • How did you get that?
  • Why did that happen?
  • Are you going to die?
  • Are you sick because of me?
  • Why do I have it?
  • What will happen to me?
  • Does it hurt?
  • Am I going to die?
  • Who else has it?
  • Why don't my brothers and sisters have it?
  • Who knows I have it?
  • Who can I tell?

Your disclosure is an ongoing process. Be open to talking with your child about hep C in the weeks following the initial disclosure. Most children take days or weeks to get up the courage to ask more questions, but parents may be so exhausted from the ordeal that they don't have the emotional energy to talk about it again. It's important to stay open to communication.

Your child will probably need to talk about his diagnosis. Assure him that he can always talk to you, and find at least one other safe, supportive person, support group, or professional counselor. If you say, "Don't tell anyone about this," he may tell someone immediately or feel resentful that he has no one to talk to. Explain what may happen if he shares this with people: telling one friend may amount to telling everyone, and some people who aren't educated about hep C may treat him badly. Expect him to be frightened when he learns he has hep C. Children of this age don't usually talk about their fears as openly as younger children, so you may have to encourage him to share his fears with you. If your child withdraws, has trouble sleeping, or experiences changes in mood or appetite, talk to him or consider seeing a counselor.

It's best not to hide your child's hep C status from her brothers and sisters. Curious peers may ask the siblings why the child is sick. It is important for the parents to minimize secrets in the home and help the siblings learn to deflect intrusive questions. Children can usually tell when something's being hidden from them. Also, if the HCV-positive child gets more attention, her siblings are less likely to be envious if they know she has a chronic disease and needs special care. Let the HCV-positive child decide if she wants to tell her siblings herself or let her parents do it. This will give her a sense of control and help her learn about telling others. If she is sick, perhaps there's something her brothers and sisters can do to help care for her. Getting them involved may help alleviate envy and teach them to be more caring and responsible. These are very fine lines for kids, and seeing a family counselor or social worker may help you learn some tips for talking to your children about disease.

Some preteens are sexually active and don't necessarily talk to their parents about it. When your child reaches the age of 10 to 13, it's important to be open about sex and sexuality and teach her about safer sex. Don't just talk about it once or give her a book. Many preteens and teenagers think of themselves as immortal, and it's important to teach them about the health and safety risks involved in all sorts of activities, including rollerblading, diving into lakes, driving, sex and foreplay, and drinking and drugs.

As your children grow up, they will want to try shaving. Be proactive and ask them if they want to shave. Buy them their own razors and beauty kits, and make sure they know not to share. Even if you don't want them to start shaving, it's better to be safe than sorry.

Teenagers

Most teenagers are curious about their bodies and have the abstract reasoning and communication skills necessary to understand the possible effects of hepatitis C and the reasons for their doctor's visits and medical treatments. They know that bad things can happen to good people, and that treatments for their disease will probably improve with future scientific research. They can also reach out for help, though they may need encouragement to do this.

The downside is that even without chronic illness, many teenagers feel different from others and are prone to feelings of alienation, depression, and low self-esteem. They are also more likely to be drinking, using drugs, having unprotected sex, and doing other things that could endanger their health, spread hep C to others, or both. Adolescence is a time when most kids want to be independent from their parents and when they feel a desperate need to fit in with their peers. Adolescents also tend to think they're immortal. It's crucial to inform your teenager that alcohol, smoking, and drugs are especially dangerous for people with hep C. But this is a delicate balancing act: your good intentions may backfire if you are too overprotective or try too hard to control your teenager's life. She will be making her own decisions about alcohol, smoking, and drugs for the rest of her life. If you acknowledge her autonomy and the fact that she's facing a lot of difficult pressures, she may be more likely to listen to you and want you to be involved in her life.

Sex and dating is confusing, anxiety ridden, and hard for teenagers, even without a chronic illness. If your teenager tells her friends she has hep C, she may have problems finding people to date. Other kids may be scared of catching hep C or of falling in love someone who is sick or could be sick sometime in the future. Your teenager is going to face many of the same relationship issues that you face as an adult. You can help him by sharing some of your own experience and listening to his. It's also important to educate him about sex. Although the rate of sexual transmission is low, make sure your teenager knows how to practice safer sex in order to prevent unwanted pregnancy and STDs, as well as hepatitis C. Depending on your teenager's age and concerns, you may want to show him or her two chapters of this book: Day 3, Telling People About Hep C, and Month 5, Yes,

You Can Have Sex, which includes a section on talking to sexual partners. If your teenager is having a particularly hard time with self-esteem and relating to peers, you may want to enlist the help of a school counselor or mental health professional.

Ultimately, parents have little control over what their adolescents learn, think, and feel. Teenagers will surf the Web and seek information from sources other than parents and doctors. While this shows curiosity and desire to learn, teenagers don't always have the knowledge and experience to weed out blatantly false information and scams—which dupe many adults as well. They may read news reports that terrify them or hear about miracle cures. Parents can be helpful by encouraging their desire to research and helping them find reliable sources of information.

Guidelines for telling a teenager about a hep C diagnosis:

○ Inform her as soon as possible.
○ Talk about the ramifications of the disease.
○ Teach standard precautions and safer sex.
○ Don't have just one conversation. The teenager will need continual emotional, intellectual, physical, and spiritual support. Ongoing discussions will help her accept the realities of hep C. Keep her informed about the disease. Encourage her to ask lots of questions and do her own research, which will give her a sense of control.
○ The teenager will want to talk to people other than his parents. Encourage him to get additional support from counselors, credible online support groups, teachers, doctors, telephone hotlines, etc.
○ The teenager will sometimes want to be treated as an adult and sometimes as a child.[6]

Disease progression and treatment in children

Children with hep C tend to experience milder symptoms than adults, and as we discussed in Month 8, studies have shown that fibrosis progresses more slowly in people who contract HCV before age 20. If your HCV-positive child is healthy, there's a good chance she won't need treatment anytime soon and can wait until more effective therapies are available.

There are currently fewer FDA-approved therapies for children with HCV than for adults. At the time this book was written, no studies had been published on treating children with pegylated interferon, but the FDA approved the use of interferon alfa-2b and ribavirin for 3- to 17-year-olds based on a study by Regino González-Peralta, M.D., and fellow researchers published in the November 2005 issue of *Hepatology*. In this relatively small study, 118 children with HCV received interferon with 15 mg/kg/day of ribavirin for 48 weeks, while other groups of children received lower doses of ribavirin. All of the children experienced side effects. Most reported mild flulike symptoms.

When the children were evaluated six months after the end of therapy, 46 percent had sustained response. This indicates that children may have a better response rate to interferon-ribavirin than adults, but the study was very small and therefore inconclusive. Children with genotypes 2 and 3 had higher response rates than children with genotype 1. Unfortunately, no African-American children received sustained response. According to the researchers, "The number of African-American children studied was too small to draw firm conclusions," but the results are consistent with data showing that African-American adults have lower response rates than other ethnic groups.[7]

The HCV-positive parent

It's a huge relief if your children test negative for HCV. But you may still have questions about being an HCV-positive parent.

O   How will I support my children if I get sick?
O   Who will take care of my children if I/we get sick?
O   I don't want my children watching me get sick.
O   What if my lifespan is significantly shortened?
O   What if I can't work?

Some parents with hepatitis C may worry that they're not good parents, especially if they experience fatigue and have difficulty participating in activities that other parents do with ease. It's important not to beat yourself up over this. If you're feeling frustrated because you don't have the energy to play with your children, you can encourage them to get involved with after-school sports, the drama club, or other activities that allow you to participate by watching and cheering your child on.

As an HCV-positive parent, you need a good support system. You may want to refer back to the section in Week 3 on building a support system. Whether or not you have a chronic illness, it's important to plan ahead in case something happens to you or you get too sick to care for your child. This is not a pleasant thought, but the more prepared you are, the less you will have to worry. You may not have much control over whether you get sick, but planning ahead is something you can control. As we discussed in Week 3, it's a good idea to know whom you can count on under what circumstances. A single mother or father with hep C may want to live close to other family members who are willing to help. If both you and your partner have hep C, this can be doubly frightening. On the one hand, you may be more capable of understanding each other's issues and difficulties. On the other hand, the fear that both of you might get sick can cause stress in your relationship. It's important that you each build your own support system and not rely on your partner alone.

Financial planning for parents

If you have hep C, one of your chief concerns may be how you're going to support your family. A chronic illness is very costly, and you may be afraid you won't be able to work. You may have to take more sick days and miss work for doctor's appointments.

Financial planning ideas for people with kids:

- ○ Make sure you and your family always have health insurance.
- ○ Look into a 401(k) or a retirement plan for when you get older.
- ○ Find out if your job offers a health plan that covers disability and future health care. Some companies offer a cancer plan, which allows you to put away money from each paycheck. Check with your human resources person to find out what you're eligible for.
- ○ Talk to a financial adviser about how you can ensure that your children will always be provided for.
- ○ Look into getting life insurance.
- ○ Consider putting money into a fund for your children in case you ever become too ill to provide for them.

If you aren't financially stable, if you freelance, or if you work at a job that doesn't offer a retirement plan or health insurance, you may want to check into government services, unions, or other organizations that can offer you some services you need. The more you plan ahead, the more control you have and the less you have to worry. Refer back to Week 2 to read more about financial planning and insurance issues.

IN A SENTENCE:

Educate your children in age-appropriate terms about preventing transmission.

Living with Coinfection

*"I've had HIV since the late 80s.
I thought I was going to die until I got on
protease inhibitors in 1996. I was doing really well
and feeling as if I could live a long life after all.
Recently my doctor gave me a test for hep C, and I
found out I have that too. Now I'm really scared.*

—NATHAN W.

*"Most people are just destroyed by the news that
they have another virus on top of HIV, but it
actually gave me hope. I was wasting away while
all my friends on protease inhibitors were doing
great, but I couldn't take the drugs they were taking
because my liver couldn't handle it. Now I know
why, and I have a doctor who believes in treating
both viruses really aggressively. I'm also really happy
about the fact that they're starting to do transplants
on HIV-positive and coinfected people.*

*I know they're just in the early stages, and it'll be years
before they're successful, but I have more treatment
options and that gives me hope."*

—JONATHAN B.

*"I had hep A before anyone even knew that hep C existed.
Years later I found out I had hep C, and that I had most
likely had hep C when I had hep A. Now I am really, really
sick with hep C, and my doctors think it is because
I had both hep A and hep C at one time."*

—MARY T.

*"I found out I was HCV-positive this year. I then went to get
an HIV test. Actually, I was so frightened that I put it off for
about six months. I wasn't sure that I wanted to know if I was
coinfected. But finally I got it. While I was waiting for the
results to come back, I couldn't even read anything about
HIV or HIV/HCV. Anytime someone came on TV talking
about HIV I got very upset. My results came back, and I was
HIV negative. I was relieved. I still have to deal with my hep
C, but not having both has given me a reason to stay clean."*

—CARLOS R.

Coinfection is a general term meaning that a person is infected with
more than one virus. It usually means that the person has HIV and HCV,
but it can also refer to coinfection with HCV and HBV or HCV and HAV.
Sometimes people talk more specifically about **dual infection** and **tri
infection:** Dual infection means that a person is infected with two viruses,
and tri infection means three viruses (most often HIV, HCV, and HBV). We
are going to focus on HCV coinfection with HIV, HBV, and HAV.

HIV disease

HIV, the human immunodeficiency virus, suppresses the immune
system by attacking the **CD4** cells. The CD4 cell, also called a **T4** and

T-helper lymphocyte, is a kind of immune cell named after a receptor on its surface. This receptor helps the CD4 cell recognize specific foreign bodies and thus fight off infection.

Until the mid-90s, there was no effective treatment for HIV. People with HIV developed opportunistic infections—infections that take advantage of a weakened immune system—such as pneumocystis carinii pneumonia (PCP), toxoplasmosis, wasting syndrome (extreme weight loss), Kaposi's sarcoma, and fungal infections. These infections frequently killed them within 10 years.

When a person tests positive for HIV antibodies and acquires certain opportunistic infections, or has a CD4 count of 200 or below, he or she is diagnosed with AIDS (acquired immunodeficiency syndrome). The term AIDS was coined in the early 80s, before scientists had discovered the HIV virus. AIDS is not the name of the virus but the name of a disease. HIV disease is a more accurate and up-to-date name, because it refers to the virus and encompasses all stages of the condition, including infection, immune suppression, and opportunistic diseases. But most people still use the term AIDS.[1]

The problem with the AIDS diagnosis is that once a person is diagnosed with AIDS, they are considered to have AIDS for the rest of their lives, even if they recover from the opportunistic infections or if their CD4 count goes up. Today, this recovery is more and more common, and the AIDS diagnosis is no longer an accurate indicator of a person's overall health or prognosis. Although people are still dying of AIDS all over the world, some effective treatments for suppressing the HIV virus were developed in the mid-90s. These treatments drastically altered the course of the disease so that some people are living much longer and have no detectable viral load. The treatments are collectively known as **highly active anti-retroviral therapies (HAART).** HAART includes reverse transcriptase inhibitors and protease inhibitors, which interfere with the replication process of HIV.

Tips for living with coinfection

Avoid alcohol

It is important that coinfected people avoid alcohol. Since HIV accelerates the progression of liver disease in patients with hep C, any alcohol may be dangerous. It is also recommended that coinfected patients consult a doctor before taking any medications or herbs.

Should I have separate health care providers?

This is one of the more important decisions you will make. It is probably better if you have one well-informed health care provider. Make sure she is up-to-date on the latest treatments and care for coinfected people. Make sure you feel comfortable with your health care provider and can be honest with her. Often friends with the same conditions can recommend good health care providers.

Here are some questions to ask when choosing a health care provider:

○ Do you have many patients with both hepatitis C and HIV?
○ How will my HIV affect my hepatitis C? How will my hepatitis C affect my HIV?
○ Are you up-to-date on the latest treatments for both HCV and HIV?
○ Do you recommend hep C treatment if I am already on an HIV treatment?
○ Do you recommend I treat my hepatitis C first before I start my HIV treatment?
○ What side effects can I expect from the medication for my HIV treatment and/or my hepatitis C treatment? What side effects can I expect taking them together?
○ Are any medications easier to take than others?
○ What changes will I have to make (diet, work schedule, social life) while I am in treatment?

IN A SENTENCE:

> *Coinfection means being infected with more than one virus, usually HCV and HIV, HBV, or HAV.*

learning

HCV with
HIV, HBV, and HAV

*"Finding out that I had HIV and HCV in one day
was the worst thing that ever happened to me.
I'd known for years that I most likely had HIV. I
was in too much denial to go get tested. As soon as
I heard about hep C, I knew I had that too.
I got the bad news all at once and knew right
away that I didn't have long to live.
There wasn't much room for false hope."*

—JEREMY P.

HIV/HCV COINFECTION has emerged as a major health problem in the last decade. In the United States alone, approximately one-third of HIV-positive people—300,000 to 400,000 people—have hepatitis C as well. Before the discovery of HAART, coinfection was less of an issue, because most coinfected people died of HIV-related causes, before their hep C had time to progress to end-stage liver disease. Many people didn't even know that they were coinfected. But now that HIV-positive people are living longer, many of them are developing severe liver disease.

Effects of HCV/HIV coinfection

HIV accelerates the course of HCV-related liver disease, but it isn't clear whether HCV affects the course of HIV. Since HIV suppresses the immune system, it may allow the hep C virus to multiply unchecked. HCV behaves as an opportunistic infection of HIV disease but is not considered an indicator of AIDS. HIV affects the immune system, making it harder for the body to fight the hepatitis C virus. The progression of liver damage may be accelerated in coinfected people, and they may be at a higher risk for cirrhosis or liver cancer. People with low CD4 cells seem to have particularly fast progression of HCV.

Highly active antiretroviral therapies (HAART) are allowing people with HIV to live much longer, making liver disease one of the top causes of death in people who are HIV/HCV coinfected. Due to the new drugs, HIV-related deaths are dropping, while HCV-related deaths (liver failure or liver cancer) are on the rise. If a patient's HIV is stable, then many doctors recommend HCV treatment. Many HAART medications are toxic to the liver, and if the HCV can be eliminated, this may reduce liver damage. The current treatment is pegylated interferon plus ribavirin. The bad news is that patients with HIV/HCV coinfection have more adverse side effects, and the therapy itself is less effective. Be aware that ribavirin should not be used with AZT, which is an ingredient in some HIV cocktails.

When the HCV protease inhibitors are approved by the FDA, it will be important to see if the HCV inhibitors interact with the HAART therapies, and to make sure HAART doesn't inhibit the HCV protease inhibitors. Hopefully, there will be a combination of HIV and HCV medications that can actually produce higher sustained response rates to HCV treatment.[3]

Liver transplants for coinfected people

Liver transplants for HIV-positive people are a promising new development on the horizon. Until very recently, people with HIV were not eligible for transplants. This was due to the fact that transplant recipients have
to take immunosuppressive drugs for the rest of their lives, and many specialists assumed that these drugs would devastate the already weakened
immune systems of HIV-positive people. It has recently been shown, however, that immunosuppressive drugs may actually slow the progress of HIV
by preventing the replication of the HIV virus. The HIV virus reproduces
by integrating itself into the DNA of T-lymphocyte immune cells. Since
immunosuppressive drugs suppress the production of immune cells, the
HIV virus cannot reproduce as quickly.

Even though liver transplants may help coinfected patients, it is often
hard for coinfected people to get transplants due to resistance on the part
of insurance companies, donor organizations, and some doctors.

Risk factors for HIV/HCV coinfection

○ Sharing IV drug needles: 50 to 90 percent of HIV-positive IV drug
   users have hep C.
○ Receiving blood products or organ transplants before the blood supply was screened for both HIV and HCV.

If you already have hep C or HIV, it's important to take preventative
measures so that you won't contract the other virus or infect someone else.
It may be easier to contract HCV if you have HIV. Moreover, coinfected
individuals appear to have higher concentrations of hep C virus in semen,
blood, and possibly other bodily fluids. HCV/HIV coinfection may make it
easier to transmit HCV both sexually and congenitally. The most important
precaution is: Don't expose yourself to blood or semen.[2]

Resources

HIV and Hepatitis.com
www.hivandhepatitis.com

Natap.org
www.natap.org

HCV/HBV coinfection

*"I shot cocaine for about six years. When I finally got clean,
I knew I had to face the music. I went to get tested and
was expecting the worst. I was sure I would have HIV.
I had never even heard of hep C. My tests came back positive
for hep C and hep B. I was relieved I didn't have HIV
but that was short-lived. Now all I do is regret what I've
done to my liver and my life."*

—ELIZABETH H.

HBV is usually not a chronic illness; it only becomes chronic in about 10 percent of people who are infected. Some studies seem to show that coinfection with HBV and HCV aggravates liver disease and can accelerate the progress of cirrhosis. It can even cause death in some people. Thus, it's really crucial to get vaccinated for hep B and hep A if you have hep C.

HCV/HAV coinfection

Some studies indicate that coinfection with hep C and hep A is life threatening because it can culminate in **fulminant hepatitis**, a sudden severe attack of hepatitis. If you have hep C you really need to get your vaccine for hep A as soon as possible.

IN A SENTENCE:

If you have hep C, it's important to get tested for HIV, HBV and HAV.

Your Future— Yes, You Have One! Why You Don't Have to Forget Your Dreams

"I told my partner Debbie I didn't want to have kids. 'Look,' I said, 'I'm 40 years old, I'm diabetic, and I have hepatitis C.' But having kids is the most important thing in Debbie's life. She told me, 'You could get hit by a truck crossing the street tomorrow, so what are we waiting for?' About a month after she got pregnant, I was diagnosed with liver cancer. It was my worst nightmare—that she'd get pregnant, and I wouldn't be there for her or the baby. I was at the top of the transplant list, but I didn't know exactly when the call would come, and they'd have an organ ready for me. I ended up having my liver transplant 11 days before Debbie had our son, Matteo. I lived through my worst nightmare. How else are you going to work through your fears?"

—JESS M.

IN A culture in which we expect to live into our 70s or 80s, a hep C diagnosis can profoundly shake up our sense of our future and our dreams. Upon receiving our diagnosis, many of us feel as if we have not yet begun to live. Most young adults in the United States expect at least four or five decades of health ahead of them and have planned their lives and careers based on this assumption.

As we said in Day 1, hepatitis C is not a death sentence. If you're relatively healthy now, you have a good chance of having a long, healthy life. The disease progresses slowly. Those of us who are infected may have an 80 percent chance of outliving hep C.

Even if you're very sick now, it's best not to forget your dreams. The will to live helps keep us alive. Many people with chronic and even terminal illnesses have outlived their doctor's prognosis simply by having a strong will to live.

> *"I had spent all my life preparing for my future. I had just finished my sixth year of medical school when I found out I had hep C. My immediate reaction was to think that my life would be much shorter now. All that time I had spent going to school, staying up all night studying, and giving up my entire life to prepare for my future had been futile. Fortunately there were a lot of doctors around whom I could talk to who knew more about hep C than I did. They explained that hep C might not affect me for decades, if at all, and that I could still realize all of my career dreams."*

—MARGARET T.

Hepatitis C can also help us focus on the present, by reminding us of our mortality. Whether or not we have hep C, none of us knows how long we'll be around, so it's important not to put our lives on hold. This doesn't mean you never have to think about the future, but you can live your life as healthily and positively as possible.

O List the things you enjoyed doing as a young child, as an older child, as an adolescent, and as a young adult. Do you still do these things? If so, try doing one of them this week, even if it feels silly. This exercise can help put you back in touch with forgotten dreams.

○ Write down your earliest and greatest dreams. Can you try doing some of them now—even on a small scale? What's preventing you? You may find, as many of us do, that the only thing standing between you and your dreams is you. You may not be able to join the ballet at 50, but perhaps you can find a place to dance, or do some kind of creative movement that's fun for you.

○ Write in your journal first thing every morning. Write whatever comes to mind without censoring yourself. The practice of journaling every morning can help you get in touch with your feelings and clear you minds of debris.

○ Find a spiritual practice or a relaxation technique that suits you and your needs. This doesn't have to involve an organized religion. Many of us find that prayer, meditation, visualization, yoga, or even relaxation CDs work wonders.

In addition to thinking about your long-term dreams and goals, you may want to make some concrete plans for your next year as well. You are now finishing your first year with hep C. You've been through a lot. It's time now to review where you've been and think about what you need to do in the next year. Taking stock of the past year can help you do this.

Review of the past year

"I was really freaked out when I was first diagnosed with hep C. I couldn't see anything good about it. But now from the perspective of a year later, I can really see some advantages. For instance, it's really made me deal with my mortality. I'm in my 20s, and I had always felt like I was immortal. It's made me realize my priorities and go after what I want. I have a much clearer sense of what I want now."

—JACK B.

This is a good time to review the journal you've been writing. Be especially sure to take a look at your first week with hep C, because that will help you appreciate how far you've come. In Day 6, Day 7, and Week 2 we focused on coming up with a plan for making necessary diet, exercise, and lifestyle changes. If you wrote this plan down in your journal, you can reevaluate where you now stand in relation to it.

Don't worry if you haven't met all your goals. Nobody's perfect. If you haven't done everything you want to do, don't beat yourself up over it. Doing 90 percent is better than doing nothing at all. The questions below may help you evaluate where you are.

○ Where are you now in terms of your level of acceptance and comfort with having hep C?
○ Where are you in achieving your goals for diet and exercise?
○ Where are you in achieving your goals for lifestyle changes?
○ If you've been following a course of treatment, how is your treatment going?
○ Do you need to reevaluate your treatment options?
○ How is your self-image?
○ Are you happy with your support system?
○ Are you happy with your doctor?
○ Are you happy with your relationships with friends, family, and your partner, if you have one?
○ Are you happy with your sex life?

If you are like most of us, chances are you haven't met all your goals. It's time to make a new schedule for the next year. At this point you may have found that some of the goals you set are not realistic or that you haven't come up with a program you can live with. The questions below may help you do this.

○ What changes do you want to make?
○ Can you live with your current diet and exercise plan?
○ Can you live with your current lifestyle changes?
○ If you are dealing with an alcohol or drug problem is your detox or recovery program working for you?
○ Do you need to try a new detox or recovery program?
○ Do you need a new doctor?
○ Do you need to get your doctor to refer you to a specialist?
○ Do you need a second opinion?

○ How is your support system working for you? Is it adequate?
○ Do you need to find more people or make more of a point of asking for what you need?

Based on what you see, can you set realistic goals for yourself for the next six months? One of the first things you can do is write down in your calendar when you need to get your liver panels in the upcoming year. You still need to get your liver panels every three months during your second year with hep C and every six months after that. You may also want to check in with your doctor and see if there are other tests that you will need this year.

> *"It's been almost a year since I was diagnosed with hep C. I've been responsible about getting my tests done. And I'm doing great. I've had a biopsy. I had some inflammation but no signs of fibrosis. I hardly have to think about hep C anymore, because the things I have to do have become second nature."*
>
> —JAMIE F.

Hopefully many of these things have become second nature, and you've been able to go on with your life. We hope our suggestions help you alleviate some symptoms you might experience or find a treatment that works for you. Hep C doesn't have to stop you from having a life. Some of us find that having hep C actually makes us more aware of our priorities. By helping us get in touch with what we really want, hep C can actually help us realize our dreams and goals.

> *"Although I decided to fight the disease, I also understood that I might not win. I began to live one day at a time, and chose to experience as much of life as I possibly could. I started trying to break down old walls between the people I love and me.*
>
> *"Now I am 24. I am a recovering addict on a maintenance program and I am living with hep C. Although I am still very scared of the possible outcome of my condition, I am also very hopeful about my future and even more determined to fight. I*

am on a waiting list to receive free treatment at St. Louis University. The program is headed by a well-known practitioner in the field, Dr. Bacon, who is said to bring about 80 percent of his patients into full remission if they start treatment in the early stages of the disease. I am, however, extremely apprehensive about getting a liver biopsy, a very painful process of extracting a piece of your liver with a long needle. But I suppose it's better than the alternative.

"It is tough sometimes, feeling self-conscious when the subject comes up or having to hide my medical status from employers and acquaintances for fear of discrimination or misguided opinions.

"Most people think that hepatitis strains are the same and contracted by being dirty or unhygienic, which I am not. I suppose that most people in my shoes would wish they hadn't been infected in the first place. And sometimes I do too. But when I think of where I might be now if I hadn't, I realize that it is for me a mixed blessing. I'm more open and honest with people than ever before. I appreciate things that otherwise I might have taken for granted. I feel urgency about life, which I didn't before. As if I've only got a finite time to accomplish my goals and do the things I want to do, so I better get moving. All in all, I feel a new sense of peace in my life that had always alluded me before. And I'm actually looking forward to new challenges. So, even though I've got a rough road ahead of me, and I'm fearful of what could happen, I'm basically grateful for what all this has given me—a brand-new outlook on life."

—ERIC CLARKSON

IN A SENTENCE:

You don't have to give up your goals and dreams just because you have hepatitis C.

learning

Keep on Learning!

ONE OF the most important things you can do for yourself in the future is to keep on learning. As you know, research on hep C is moving at a furious pace. We've tried to give you a lot of background information, so that you can understand the terminology in various papers and articles on hep C and discuss your condition intelligently with your doctor. In Month 7, we've given you some tools to do research on your own. We encourage you to review this chapter and to use the resource section in the back of this book. We've compiled a wealth of resources, including liver organizations, publications, Web sites, chat rooms, newsgroups, and various sources of information on conventional, complementary, and alternative treatments. We hope that these resources will serve you well for a long time.

Our greatest wish for you and for all of us is that scientists will soon discover a cure for hepatitis C. While we're waiting, we hope that you'll continue to learn to live with this chronic, yet manageable, illness. We also hope that your health care becomes second nature to such an extent that you hardly have to think about it.

Good luck!

IN A SENTENCE:

> *Research is moving at a furious pace: Keep learning!*

Glossary

ACUPUNCTURE: in traditional Chinese medicine, the practice of inserting fine needles into specific points on the body in order to change the flow of Qi ("energy").

ALBUMIN: a blood protein produced by the liver. Albumin maintains the volume of blood in blood vessels by absorbing fluid (salt and water). Low albumin level may cause fluid to leak out of arteries and veins into tissues and cause swelling, called **edema**.

ALKALINE PHOSPHATASE (ALK): a liver enzyme that activates the metabolism of phosphorus and delivers energy to cells in the body. Abnormal ALK may indicate bile duct blockage or alcohol or drug induced hepatitis.

ALT (ALANINE AMINOTRANSFERASE) AND AST (ASPARTATE AMINOTRANSFERASE): a common test used to monitor liver damage in people who have hepatitis C. ALT and AST are enzymes used for the metabolism of amino acids. Liver cells release these enzymes into the bloodstream when they die. Elevated enzymes indicate inflammation and possibly HCV.

ANECDOTAL EVIDENCE: evidence based on the reports of individuals, rather than scientific studies.

ANTIBODIES: proteins that fight infections. Antibodies fit into molecules (called **antigens**) on the surface of the virus like a key fits into a lock. Once antibodies attach to the virus's surface, the body's white blood cells can locate the virus and fight the infection.

ANTI-HCV ANTIBODY TEST: a test to see if you have antibodies to the HCV virus. A "positive" or "reactive" test indicates that you have been exposed to HCV, and your body has mounted a defense by producing antibodies. The antibody test indicates past or present infection. It does not indicate whether the virus is present in your body. Even if your body has successfully eliminated HCV, this test will still be positive.

ANTI-HCV ELISA 3 (ENZYME-LINKED IMMUNOSORBENT ASSAY) OR EIA (ENZYME IMMUNOASSAY): the most widely used test for HCV antibodies.

ANTIOXIDANTS: substances that prevent a process called oxidation, which can corrode tissues such as blood vessel walls and liver cells. Oxidized liver cells are more susceptible to cirrhosis and cancer. Free radicals are substances that can cause oxidation. Antioxidants intercept free radicals and prevent the process of oxidation.

ASCITES: fluid retention in the abdomen, may be a symptom of severe liver disease. The swelling of the **portal vein** can block the lymph channels and cause lymph to spill into the abdomen, causing **ascites**, swelling of the abdomen, and sometimes **edema**, swelling of the legs.

AST (ASPARTATE AMINOTRANSFERASE): see **ALT.**

ASYMPTOMATIC: having no symptoms.

AUTOIMMUNE HEPATITIS: inflammation of the liver caused by the immune system attacking liver cells.

AYURVEDA: ("knowledge of life") the national health care system of India and Sri Lanka.

BILE: The liver produces and secretes bile, a yellow-green fluid, which helps your body digest food and absorb nutrients. Bile, also called gall, contains water, bile pigments like **bilirubin**, bile acids and salts, fatty acids, and cholesterol. After the liver produces bile, the gallbladder acts as reservoir, storing bile and releasing it into the small intestine. Bile salts liquefy fats, so that they can be digested by the enzymes in the intestines. **Jaundice** develops when bile, which usually passes from the liver to the intestines, gets blocked and overflows into the body and builds up in the skin.

BILIARY TRACT: the ducts that drain bile from the liver into the intestine.

BILIRUBIN: a yellowish pigment produced in the breakdown of red blood cells. This breakdown first produces hemoglobin, and its major component is converted into **bilirubin**. The liver recycles bilirubin into **bile**. A high level of bilirubin may indicate that too many red blood cells are dying. The buildup of bilirubin in the skin causes **jaundice**, a common symptom of hepatitis A and B.

BIOPSY: See **liver biopsy.**

BLEEDING VARICES: may be a symptom of severe liver disease. "Varices" are swollen veins—like varicose veins, only they're inside the body. When blood gets backed up in the **portal vein**, blood vessels in the esophagus and stomach can also swell. These swollen veins may begin leaking blood.

CADAVERIC TRANSPLANT: a term used in the context of organ transplantation; a transplant in which the new organ comes from someone who has recently died.

CAPSID: scientific word for the protein coat encasing a virus.

CD4 AND CD8: CD4 and CD8 are "membrane glycoproteins," on the surface of immune system cells called T-lymphocytes, a type of white blood cell. These "membrane glycoproteins" determine how the cell recognizes specific foreign bodies and fights off infection. The HIV virus weakens the immune system by attacking the CD4 cells. CD4 cells are also called T4 and T-helper lymphocytes.

CHRONIC HEPATITIS: hepatitis lasting more than six months.

CIRRHOSIS: (means "scarring") scarring so extensive that it changes the structure and function of the liver. Chronic hepatitis, or chronic inflammation of the liver, can hinder the circulation of blood through the liver and cause liver cells to die. These dead cells harden, forming scar tissue on the liver. This buildup of fibrous scar tissue is called **fibrosis.** When fibrosis is so extensive it distorts the liver's structure and function, it becomes **cirrhosis**.

COAGULOPATHY: disturbances in blood clotting. People with this condition may bruise extremely easily and bleed profusely with minor cuts. Coagulopathy most often results from the liver being unable to make certain clotting factors from vitamin K.

COINFECTION: a general term meaning that a person is infected with more than one virus. It usually means that the person has HIV and HCV, but it can also refer to coinfection with HCV and HBV or HCV and HAV.

COMBINATION THERAPY: the combination of interferon and ribavirin used to treat hepatitis.

COMPENSATED CIRRHOSIS: cirrhosis without symptoms.

CONGENITAL TRANSMISSION: transmission of a disease from mother to child during pregnancy or the birth process.

CONTRAINDICATION: an indication that it's not advisable (e.g., to combine one treatment with another).

CONTROLLED STUDY: a study in which some of the participants receive the drug that is being studied, and others (the "control group") take a placebo, a pill that doesn't contain the medication. The participants don't know whether they're getting the drug or not. In a "double blind" study their doctors don't know either. The purpose of the control group is to tell whether the medication is having an effect. It's possible that the people would get better anyway, or that they would get better because they believed that the drug would cure them.

CORE-POSITIVE ORGAN: a term used in the context of liver transplantation. If an organ tests positive for HCV or HBV, it is called a core-positive organ, and it can be transplanted into someone who tests positive for HCV or HBV.

CRYOGLOBULINEMIA: a condition that can be related to hep C; an immune disturbance, caused by immunoglobin, a type of antibody that the body produces to combat HCV. In this condition, proteins may clump together in the blood and damage the skin, nervous system, kidneys, eyes, brain and heart. When this clustering occurs in the part of the kidney that filters blood (the glomerulus), it may cause plugging, which can damage the membrane and sometimes lead to kidney failure. Cryoglobulinemia may also cause intense itching, which can be uncomfortable and difficult to live with.

CT (COMPUTERIZED TOMOGRAPHY) SCAN: a nonintrusive procedure used for evaluating damage to the liver; not as precise as the biopsy, but more detailed than an ultrasound. Low-level radiation offers an image of a cross section of a person's body.

CULTURE: To "culture" a virus means to grow it outside the human body in a laboratory.

CYSTEINE: an amino acid that helps the body make glutathione, which plays a major role in the liver's detoxification process.

CYTOPLASM: the solution inside a cell surrounding the nucleus.

DECOMPENSATED CIRRHOSIS: Cirrhosis with symptoms, in contrast to "compensated" or asymptomatic cirrhosis.

DETOX: short for "detoxification," process of eliminating toxins from the body; often refers to the process of quitting drugs or alcohol.

DIURETICS: water pills that make you urinate.

DNA (DEOXYRIBONUCLEIC ACID): One of the main types of nucleic acids, DNA is responsible for carrying an organism's genetic information to its offspring. DNA is the molecule inside the nucleus of a cell that encodes genetic information and determines the cell's behavior, structure, and functions.

DUAL INFECTION: type of coinfection in which a person is infected with two viruses.

EDEMA: swelling of the legs, may be a symptom of severe liver disease. The swelling of the **portal vein** can block the lymph channels and cause lymph to spill into the abdomen, causing edema, as well as **ascites**. Low albumin level may also cause fluid to leak out of arteries and veins into tissues and cause edema.

ELISA 3: See Anti-HCV ELISA 3.

ENCEPHALOPATHY: may be a symptom of severe liver disease. Cognitive and personality changes and neurologic disorders, due to the buildup of ammonia and other toxins. Mild encephalopathy is characterized by lethargy, disorientation, and tremor. Severe cases may lead to coma.

ENZYMES: proteins that make particular chemical reactions happen.

FIBROSIS: formation of fibrous scar tissue on the liver. Chronic hepatitis, or chronic inflammation of the liver, can hinder the circulation of blood through the liver and cause liver cells to die. These dead cells harden, forming scar tissue on the liver. This buildup of fibrous scar tissue is called **fibrosis.** When fibrosis is so extensive it distorts the liver's structure and function, it becomes **cirrhosis**.

FREE RADICALS: substances that can cause oxidation. Oxidation is a chemical process that can corrode tissues such as blood vessel walls and liver cells. Oxidized liver cells are more susceptible to cirrhosis and cancer. Antioxidants intercept free radicals and prevent the process of oxidation.

FULMINANT HEPATITIS: a sudden severe attack of hepatitis.

GAMMA-GLUTAMYL TRANSPEPTIDASE (GGT): an enzyme that helps in the metabolism of glutamate.

GASTROENTEROLOGIST: a physician who specializes in disorders of the stomach and intestines.

GENOME: a virus's or organism's genetic material.

GENOTYPES: genetic variations.

GLOMERULUS: the part of the kidney that filters blood.

HCV: the virus that causes hepatitis C.

HCV RNA: hepatitis C virus ribonucleic acid; the genetic material of the HCV virus. The PCR test detects the presence of the virus by detecting HCV RNA in the blood.

HEME: the main component of hemoglobin. An enzyme called heme oxygenase converts heme into **bilirubin**.

HEMOGLOBIN: a molecule that carries oxygen in red blood cells to the tissues in the body.

HEMORRHAGIC STROKE. A stroke caused by a blood vessel in the brain leaking blood into brain tissue. The underlying cause is usually a malformed blood vessel or high blood pressure.

HEPATITIS: inflammation of the liver.

HEPATOCELLULAR CARCINOMA (HCC): liver cancer.

HEPATOLOGIST: a physician who specializes in the liver.

HIV (HUMAN IMMUNODEFICIENCY VIRUS): the virus that causes HIV disease. HIV impairs the immune system by infecting the immune cells, particularly the T lymphocytes.

HOLISTIC TREATMENT: a treatment that emphasizes the whole person rather than the parts.

HOMEOPATHY: the practice of treating an illness by giving the patient a tiny dose of a substance that produces effects similar to the symptoms of the disease. This contrasts with conventional western or "allopathic" medicine, which prescribes medications that produce effects different from the disease. (*Homeo* means "same," while *allo* means "other.")

HYPOTHROIDISM: the reduced production of thyroid hormones.

HYPERTHYROIDISM: the increased production of thyroid hormones.

INTERFERON: When a virus invades one of our cells, that cell produces proteins called interferons, which cause the cells around it to produce enzymes that hopefully stop the virus from replicating. Drug companies have produced synthetic interferons, some of which have been approved for treating hepatitis C, as well as other diseases.

IV: intravenous, meaning "into the vein." IV needles or syringes are used to inject substances into a vein.

IVDU: stands for "intravenous drug user."

JAUNDICE: a common symptom of hepatitis A and B; yellow skin and eyes, due to inadequate processing of bilirubin, which builds up in the skin.

JAUNDICE PRURITIS: Intense itching caused by **jaundice.**

LIVER BIOPSY: the most widely used tool for diagnosing and evaluating liver damage; a relatively simple surgical procedure, where the doctor inserts a needle between your ribs, extracts 1/50,000th of the liver, and examines the tissue under a microscope to see if fibrosis or cirrhosis is present. The grade of inflammation and the stage of fibrosis are measured on two separate scales from 0 to 4.

LIVER TRANSPLANT SURGERY: the process of removing a liver that no longer functions and replacing it with a healthier liver taken from the body of an organ donor.

LIVING DONOR LIVER TRANSPLANT: a surgical procedure in which 60 percent to 70 percent of a living person's liver is removed and put into the body of someone who needs a liver. Since the liver can regenerate 3/4 of its tissue in a few weeks, both the donor and recipient have fully functioning livers a few months after the operation.

MUTATIONS: small changes in genetic material.

OXIDATION: a chemical process that can corrode tissues such as blood vessel walls and liver cells. Oxidized liver cells are more susceptible to cirrhosis and cancer. Free radicals are substances that can cause oxidation. Antioxidants intercept free radicals and prevent the process of oxidation

PARACENTESIS: procedure in which a physician sticks a needle into the body to draw out fluid, such as **ascites.**

PASSIVE TRANSFER: a process in which antibodies to hep C cross the mother's placental barrier and become detectable in the fetus's blood. These antibodies usually remain detectable for a period of three to six months after birth, They do not indicate whether or not the child is infected with hep C. Unfortunately they don't prevent the child from contracting hep C either. If the antibodies are still detectable after one year, the child is diagnosed with chronic hepatitis C.

PCR TEST (POLYMERASE CHAIN REACTION): a test used to confirm that the virus is present in your bloodstream. The test measures **HCV RNA**, the genetic material of the virus, and your **viral load**, the number of copies of the virus in one milliliter of blood.

PEGYLATED INTERFERON: time release interferon. Pegylation is the process of adding a molecule of polyethylene glycol to interferon. The polyethylene glycol acts like a suit of armor—making the interferon time release and increasing absorption, so that patients only have to inject the interferon once a week, rather than three times a week. This pharmaceutical is thought to have less severe side effects than regular interferon.

PERINATAL TRANSMISSION: transmission of a disease from mother to child during pregnancy or the birth process.

PORTAL HYPERTENSION: High blood pressure in the portal vein. When blood cannot flow freely through the liver, it collects in the portal vein, and pressure builds, causing the vein to swell. This exerts pressure on the surrounding organs and causes the heart to work harder.

PORTAL VEIN: vein that collects blood from organs in the abdomen, including the stomach and intestines, and transports this blood to the liver.

PROTEASE INHIBITORS: antivirals that bind to specific sites on a virus and halt viral replication; currently used in treating HIV.

PROTHROMBIN TIME (PT): Prothrombin is a protein that helps the blood clot. The test for **prothrombin time** measures how long the blood takes to clot. When the liver is not functioning well, blood clotting as measured by PT may be slower, and the person will bleed and bruise easily.

PRURITIS: Intense itching. See **jaundice pruritis.**

RANDOMIZED DOUBLE-BLIND PLACEBO-CONTROLLED (RDBPC) STUDY: This kind of study is considered most scientifically rigorous for establishing the safety and effectiveness of a new kind of treatment. In an RDBPC study, participants are randomly divided into two groups. Some of the participants receive the drug that is being studied, and others (the "control group") take a placebo, a pill that doesn't contain the medication. The participants don't know whether they're getting the drug or not. The study is called "double blind" because their doctors don't know either. The purpose of the control group is to tell whether the medication is having an effect: it's possible that the people would get better anyway, or that they would get better because they believed that the drug would cure them.

RECOMMENDED DAILY ALLOWANCE (USRDA): See **reference daily intake (RDI).**

REFERENCE DAILY INTAKE (RDI): used to be called the **recommended daily allowance (USRDA);** the minimum amounts of vitamins and minerals you need on a daily basis to avoid vitamin and mineral deficiencies, such as rickets and scurvy.

REPLICATION: the way a virus reproduces by copying its genetic material.

RHEUMATOID ARTHRITIS: a condition characterized by joint pain and swelling, sometimes related to hep C.

RIBA 3 (RECOMBINANT IMMUNOBLOT ASSAY): Test for HCV antibodies used to verify a positive result on the less accurate ELISA 3.

RIBAVIRIN: a pharmaceutical drug that may slow the genetic machinery of the HCV virus and may also help preserve some immune functions; used in combination with interferon to treat hepatitis C.

RNA (RIBONUCLEIC ACID): One of the main types of nucleic acids, RNA delivers the information coded in DNA to the ribosome, the factory inside the cell that synthesizes proteins. Some viruses, like hep C, contain only RNA and not DNA.

SEROCONVERSION: the body's process of mounting an immune response and producing antibodies to a virus. At the end of this process, the patient tests positive for the virus; the period between the initial exposure and the point at which laboratory tests indicate the presence of antibodies in the blood.

SILYMARIN: the ingredient in milk thistle that supposedly protects the liver.

SPONTANEOUS BACTERIAL PERITONITIS: a bacterial infection in the abdomen, requiring antibiotic treatment.

STANDARD PRECAUTIONS: The CDC's guidelines for preventing the transmission of blood-borne pathogens, such as hep C, HIV and hep B. These precautions involve wearing latex or polyurethane gloves when you come into contact with any body fluid except sweat, unless you can easily contain the fluid with a thick cloth or nonporous material.

STD (SEXUALLY TRANSMITTED DISEASE): a disease primarily transmitted through sexual contact.

STERILIZATION: the process of destroying all microbial life. Sterilization is usually done in a hospital through moist heat by steam autoclaving, ethylene oxide gas, and dry heat.

SUBCUTANEOUS: "under the skin," injected under the skin, as with a syringe.

SUSTAINED VIRAL RESPONSE (SVR): the patient has an undetectable viral load (HCV RNA) six months following treatment.

THROMBOCYTOPENIA: a condition characterized by low blood platelets, which are needed for clotting.

TMA (TRANSCRIPTION MEDIATED AMPLIFICATION): a highly sensitive viral load test that can detect few as 50 copies of HCV virus in one milliliter of blood.

TRANS-FATS: a fat that is made to be solid at room temperature, such as margarine.

TRI INFECTION: type of coinfection in which a person is infected with three viruses (most often HIV, HCV, and HBV).

ULTRASOUND SCAN: a nonintrusive procedure used for evaluating damage to the liver; not as precise as the biopsy. The ultrasound machine translates sound waves that bounce off your organs into visual images, which can show the liver's structure and condition and detect the growth of tumors and changes in the portal vein and hepatic artery.

VACCINE: subcutaneous injection of dead viruses into the body. The body's immune system produces **antibodies** to the virus, so the person is immune to the disease.

VERTICAL TRANSMISSION: transmission of a disease from mother to child.

VIRAL LOAD: the quantity of virus in the blood; more specifically, the number of copies of the virus in one milliliter of blood.

VIRUS: a capsule (called "**capsid**"), containing strands of genetic material, made up of nucleic acids and proteins. Unlike bacteria, they have no metabolism and none of the other systems that support life. All they do is replicate, but they need to occupy the cells of a living organism (a "host") in order to do this. The hep C virus is a parasite, and you are the host that the virus needs to replicate itself.

WORKS: IV drug paraphernalia. This equipment may include syringes (IV needles), spoons, tourniquets (or "ties"), "cookers" (spoons or anything used to "cook" drugs), and water.

Notes

Introduction

1. Estimates differ widely, ranging from 200 to 300 million. The 300
   million estimate appears in many sources, including the following
   study in the January 2006 issue of *Hepatology*, the official journal of
   the American Association of the Study of Liver Diseases (AASLD):
   Yoshiaki Iwasaki, et al. "Limitation of combination therapy of
   interferon and ribavirin for older patients with chronic hepatitis C."
   Hepatology, January 2006 (DOI: 10.1002/hep.20984)
   www.interscience.wiley.com/journal/hepatology; cited in "Difficulty
   In treating older hepatitis C patients with combination therapy."
   www.medicalnewstoday.com/medicalnews.php?
   newsid=35854

2. Estimates vary as to what percent of IV drug users are infected with
   hep C. Melissa Palmer, M.D. says 85 to 100 percent; the *American
   Journal of Epidemiology* says 70 to 90 percent of current IV drug
   users are infected, with as many as 95 percent after five years of
   using. The National Institute on Drug Abuse (NIDA) says hepatitis
   C infection happens very soon as initiation into injection drug use
   begins: 50 to 80 percent contract the virus within 6 to 12 months.

Day 1

1. Elisabeth Kübler-Ross, M.D., *On Death and Dying* (New York:
   Macmillan, 1969).

2. M.G. Pessoa, M.D., N.A. Terrault, M.D. J. Detmer, M.D; J.M. Kolberg, M.D; M. Collins, M.D; H.M. Hassoba, M.D; T.L. Wright, M.D. "Quantitation of hepatitis G and C viruses in the liver: evidence that hepatitis G virus is not hepatotropic." *Hepatology* 1998 Mar; 27(3):877–80.

R. Halasz, M.D. M. Sallberg, M.D., S. Lundholm, M.D., G. Andersson, M.D., B. Lager, M.D., H. Glaumann, M.D., O. Weiland, M.D., "The GB virus C/hepatitis G virus replicates in hepatocytes without causing liver disease in healthy blood donors," *Journal of Infectious Disease* 2000 Dec; 182(6): 1756–60.

3. Matthew Dolan, author of *The Hepatitis C Handbook,* discussed the work of Peter Simmonds, Ph.D. and the history of how Hepatitis C spread throughout the world in a lecture entitled "Hepatitis C: A Global Perspective." Fifth International Hepatitis C Conference, Hepatitis C Global Foundation, Holiday Inn, Golden Gateway, San Francisco, 3 August 2001.

4. "National Institutes of Health Consensus Development Conference Statement: Management of hepatitis C 2002" (June 10–12, 2002). *Gastroenterology.* 2002;123(6):2082–99.

5. "Hepatitis C," in PKIDs (Parents of Kids with Infectious Diseases), *Pediatric Hepatitis Report,* pp. 123-4. Hepatitis C Council of New South Wales, "Genotypes." www.hepatitisc.org.au/quickref/documents/Genotypes.pdf

Day 2

1. In a recent German study, 44 patients, who had been infected with hep C for an average of 89 days, were treated with 5 million U of interferon alpha-2b daily for 4 weeks, then three times per week the following 20 weeks. At 24 weeks following the end of treatment, 42 of the patients had no detectable hep C viral RNA in their blood. Elmar Jaeckel, M.D., Markus Cornberg, M.D., Heiner Wedemeyer, M.D., Teresa Santantonio, M.D., Julika Mayer, M.D., Myrga Zankel, D.V.M., Giuseppe Pastore, M.D., Manfred Dietrich, M.D., Christian Trautwein, M.D., Michael P. Manns, M.D., and the German Acute Hepatitis C Therapy Group, "Treatment of Acute Hepatitis C with Interferon Alpha-2b," *New England Journal of Medicine,* November 15, 2001. See www. nejm.org, October 1, 2001.

2. See the following studies.

S. Anderson, M.D., C.L. Nevins, M.D., L.K. Green M.D., H. El-Zimaity, M.D., B.S. Anand, M.D., "Assessment of liver histology in chronic alcoholics with and without hepatitis C virus infection," *Digestive Disease Sciences* 2001 Jul; 46(7):1393–8.

G. Corrao, M.D., S. Arico, M.D., "Independent and combined action of hepatitis C virus infection and alcohol consumption on the risk of symptomatic liver cirrhosis," *Hepatology* 1998 Apr; 27(4): 914–9.

D.R. Harris, R. Gonin, H.J. Alter, E.C. Wright, Z.J. Buskell, F.B. Hollinger, L.B. Seeff. "The relationship of acute transfusion-associated hepatitis to the development of cirrhosis in the presence of alcohol abuse." *Ann Intern Med* 2001 Jan 16; 134(2): 120–4.

C.L.Nevins, M.D., H. Malaty, M.D., M.E. Velez, M.D., B.S. Anand, M.D., "Interaction of alcohol and hepatitis C virus infection on severity of liver disease," *Dig Dis Sci* 1999 Jun;44(6):1236–42.

Ostapowicz, M.D., Watson, M.D., Locarnini, M.D., Desmond, M.D., "Role of alcohol in the progression of liver disease caused by hepatitis C virus infection," *Hepatology* 1998 Jun; 27(6): 1730–5.

Pessione, M.D., Degos, M.D., Marcellin, M.D., Duchatelle, M.D., Njapoum, M.D., Martinot-Peignoux, M.D., Degott, M.D., Valla, M.D., Erlinger, M.D., Rueff, M.D., "Effect of alcohol consumption on serum hepatitis C virus RNA and histological lesions in chronic hepatitis C," *Hepatology* 1998 Jun; 27(6):1717–22.

Chen, Stephen L. and Timothy R. Morgan. "The natural history of hepatitis C virus (HCV) infection." *International Journal of Medical Science*. 2006; 3(2): 47–52, www.pubmedcentral.nih.gov/articlerender.fcgi?artid=1415841#top

Wiley T.E. et al. Impact of alcohol on the histological and clinical progression of hepatitis C infection. *Hepatology*.1998;28(3):805–9.

Noda, K. et al. Progression of type C chronic hepatitis to liver cirrhosis and hepatocellular carcinoma—its relationship to alcohol drinking and the age of transfusion. *Alcohol Clin* Exp Res. 1996;20(1 Suppl):95A–100A.

Peters, M. G, Terrault N. A. "Alcohol use and hepatitis C." *Hepatology*. 2002;36(5 Suppl 1):S220–5.

Poynard T, Bedossa P, Opolon P. "Natural history of liver fibrosis progression in patients with chronic hepatitis C." The OBSVIRC, METAVIR, CLINIVIR, and DOSVIRC groups. *Lancet*. 1997;349(9055):825–32.

3. Wenzhe Ho, Steven D. Douglas, and colleagues report their results in *Hepatology*, July 2003; 38:1, 57–65; www.niaaa.nih.gov/NewsEvents/NewsReleases/hepatitis.htm

4. National Institutes of Health Consensus Development Conference Statement: Management of hepatitis C 2002 (June 10–12, 2002). *Gastroenterology*. 2002;123(6):2082–99.

5. CDC. "Frequently asked questions about hepatitis C." December 2006. www.cdc.gov.mill1.sjlibrary.org/ncidod/diseases/hepatitis/c/faq.htm#1b1

6. PKIDs (Parents of Kids With Infectious Diseases). "Standard Precautions Stop the Spread of Infections in Daily Life." *Pediatric Hepatitis Report*, pp. 283-6; http://www.pkids.org/pdf/phr/08-04stdprecautions.pdf

Day 3

1. Steckelberg, James, M.D. "How common is sexual transmission?" Mayo Clinic. www.mayoclinic.com/health/hepatitis-c/AN00701

Day 4

1. National Institutes of Health. "Chronic Hepatitis C: Current Disease Management." National Institute of Diabetes and Digestive and Kidney Diseases (NIDDK) November 2006. http://digestive.niddk.nih.gov/ddiseases/pubs/chronichepc/index.htm

Day 6

1. Palmer, p. 344.

2. Klatsky, A. et al. "Coffee, cirrhosis, and transaminase enzymes." *Archives of Internal Medicine*. June 12, 2006; vol 166: pp. 1190–1195.

3. Corrao, G. et al. "The effect of drinking coffee and smoking cigarettes on the risk of cirrhosis associated with alcohol consumption." *European Journal of Epidemiology*. 1994. Dec;10(6): 657–664.

   Corrao, G. et al. "Coffee, caffeine, and the risk of liver cirrhosis." *Annals of Epidemiology*. Oct 2001;11(7): 458–465.

   Gallus, S. et al. "Does coffee protect against liver cirrhosis?" *Annals of Epidemiology*. Apr 2002;12(3): 202–205.

4. Armstrong, L.E. *International Journal of Sport Nutrition and Exercise Metabolism*. 2002, 12; 189–206.

Day 7

1. Erowid. "Cannabis Basics."
   www.erowid.org/plants/cannabis/cannabis_basics.shtml#problems

2. Beitia, G., Cobreros, A., Sainz, L., Cenarruzabeitia, E. "MDMA (ecstasy)-induced hepatoxicity; effect on cytosolic calcium signals in isolated hepatocytes." *Liver* 1999; 19(3):234–41. www.erowid.org/references/refs_view.php?ID=259

   Carvalho, M., Carvalho, F., and Bastos, M. L. "Is hyperthermia the triggering factor for the hepatoxicity induced by 3,4-methylenedioxymethamphetamine (ecstasy)? An in vitro study using freshly isolated mouse hepatocytes." *Arch Toxicol* 2001; 74:789–93. www.erowid.org/references/refs_view.php?ID=1143

   Carvalho, M., Carvalho, F., Remiao, F., de Lourdes Pereira, M., Pires-Das-Neves, R., de Lourdes Bastos, M. "Effect of 3,4-methylenedioxymethamphetamine ('ecstasy') on body temperature and liver antioxidant status in mice: influence of ambient temperature." *Arch Toxicol* 2002; 76(3):166–172. www.erowid.org/references/refs_view.php?ID=1383

3. *Shroomery*. "Do hallucinogenic mushrooms cause liver damage?" Magic Mushrooms Demystified. www.shroomery.org/8763/Do-hallucinogenic-mushrooms-cause-liver-damage

4. Cox, Audra. "Hepatitis C complicated by morphine withdrawal." *Medical News Today*. 2005. www.medicalnewstoday.com/medicalnews.php?newsid=32798

   Johnson, Carla K. "High Tylenol doses linked to liver woes." Associated Press. July 2006. www.washtimes.com/national/20060704-115220-4848r.htm
   UIC College of Pharmacy. "Use of pain medications in hepatic insufficiency." www.uic.edu/pharmacy/services/di/liver.htm

   Yuan Li, Ting Zhang, Steven D. Douglas, Jian-Ping Lai, Wei-Dong Xiao, David E. Pleasure, Wen-Zhe Ho. "Morphine enhances hepatitis C (HCV) replicon expression." *American Journal of Pathology*, 2003. 163:1167–1175. ajp.amjpathol.org/cgi/content/full/163/3/1167

5. Sylvestre, D. L. "Treating hepatitis C in methadone maintenance patients: an interim analysis." *Drug Alcohol Depend.* July 2002. 67(2): 117–23. www.ncbi.nlm.nih.gov/entrez/query.fcgi?cmd=Retrieve&db=PubMed&list_uids= 12095661&dopt=Abstract

Edlin, B. "Prevention and treatment of hepatitis C in injection drug users." *Hepatology.* November 2002. 36(5 Suppl. 1): S210–9. www.pubmedcentral.nih.gov/articlerender.fcgi?artid=1629041

Mauss, S. et al. "A prospective controlled study of interferon-based therapy of chronic hepatitis C in patients on methadone maintenance." *Hepatology.* July 2004. 40 (1): 120–124. www.ncbi.nlm.nih.gov/entrez/query.fcgi?cmd=Retrieve&db=PubMed&list_uids= 15239094&dopt=Abstract

Verrando, R., Robaeys, G., Mathei, C., Buntinx, F. "Methadone and buprenorphine maintenance therapies for patients with hepatitis C virus infected after intravenous drug use." *Acta Gastroenterol Belg.* Jan—Mar, 2005: 68(1):81–5. www.ncbi.nlm.nih.gov/entrez/query.fcgi?cmd=Retrieve&db =PubMed&list_uids=15832591&dopt=Abstract

Herve, S., Riachi, G., Noblet, C., Guillement, N., et al. "Acute hepatitis due to buprenorphine administration." *Eur J Gastroenterol Hepatol.* Oct 2004: 16(10): 1033–7. www.ncbi.nlm.nih.gov/entrez/query.fcgi?cmd=Retrieve&db= PubMed&list_uids=15371928&dopt=Abstract

Morrill, James A., M.D., PhD., Shrestha, M., B.S., CHES., Grant, Richard W., M.D., MPH. "Barriers to the treatment of hepatitis C: Patient, provider, and system factors." *J Gen Intern Med.* 2005 August; 20(8): 754–758. www.pubmedcentral.nih.gov/articlerender.fcgi?artid=1490173

Trocho, C. "The Barcelona Report." www.presidiotex.com/barcelona/

Lee, Dennis. "Drug Induced liver disease." Medicine Net. 2006. www.medicinenet.com/drug_induced_liver_disease/article.htm

Week 2

1. The Association of Healthcare Journalists. "Chronic Illness: Treatment without cure. Can the system cope?" *Covering the Quality of Healthcare: A Resource Guide for Journalists* 2002. www.healthjournalism.org/qualityguide/ chapter3.html

Chambers, Jacques. "Guarantee Issue Health Insurance." HCVAdvocate.org. 2003. hcvadvocate.org/hepatitis/hepc/guarantee_insurance.html

"State Coverage Initiatives." Academy Health. statecoverage.net.

U.S. Census Bureau. "Income, Poverty and Health Insurance Coverage in the United States: 2004." August 2005. www.census.gov/prod/2005pubs/ p60–229.pdf

U.S. Department of Labor. "Health plans and benefits." January 2007. www.dol.gov/dol/topic/health-plans/index.htm

Partnership for Solutions. "Better lives for people with chronic conditions." 2001. www.partnershipforsolutions.org

Week 4

1. Melissa Palmer, M.D. *Dr. Melissa Palmer's Guide to Hepatitis and Liver Disease: What You Need to Know.* Revised Edition. (Avery 2004) p. 144.

2. Palmer, pp. 146–159, 316–318, 425.

3. Palmer, pp. 191–5.

4. Schering-Plough. "PEG-INTRON(R) and REBETOL(R) combination therapy demonstrates consistently high response rates across patient weight groups in 'real-life' treatment setting." www.schering-plough.com/schering_plough/news/release.jsp?releaseID=782099

5. V. J. Smith, R.N., B.S.N., M.A. "How durable is the HCV sustained viral response?" National AIDS Treatment Advocacy Project (NATAP). August 2004. www.natap.org/2004/HCV/083004_06.htm

Month 2

1. Liu, J., Manheimer, E., Tsutani, K., et al. "Medicinal herbs for hepatitis C virus infection: a Cochrane hepatobiliary systematic review of randomized trials." *The American Journal of Gastroenterology.* 2003;98(3):538–544.

2. PKIDs. "CAM: Complementary and Alternative Medicines." *Pediatric Hepatitis Report,* p. 6. www.pkids.org/pdf/phr/08-06cam.pdf

3. Palmer, p. 345.

4. PKIDs. "CAM: Complementary and Alternative Medicines." *Pediatric Hepatitis Report,* p. 9. www.pkids.org/pdf/phr/08-06cam.pdf

Month 3

1. Highleyman, Liz. "HCV continues to replicate in the livers of patients with sustained response to therapy." www.hivandhepatitis.com/hep_c/news/2007/121506_b.html

2. National Institutes of Health. "New in vitro model system will allow study of therapeutics and virus life cycle." National Institute of Diabetes and Digestive and Kidney Diseases (NIDDK), Press Release. February 22, 2005. www.niddk.nih.gov/welcome/releases/02-22-05.htm

   Heller, Theo; Jonathan Auerbach; Tarice Williams; Tzivia Rachel Moreen; Allison Jazwinski; Brian Cruz; Neha Jeurkar; Ronda Sapp; Guangxiang Luo; and T. Jake Liang. "An in vitro model of hepatitis C virion production." *Proceedings of the National Academy of Sciences,* Vol. 102, No. 7, pp. 2579–2583.

3. Hepatitis Central. "Novel virus culture system for hepatitis C." Hepatitis C Information Center, February 2, 2007. hepatitis-central.com/mt/archives/2007/02/novel_virus_cul.html

4. Gish, Robert G. "Future therapies." *HCV Advocate,* Feb. 2006. www.hcvadvocate.org/hcsp/articles/Future_therapies.html

5. Highleyman, Liz. "AASLD: Investigational antiviral therapies for hepatitis C." *HCV Advocate Newsletter*, Dec. 2006. www.hcvadvocate.org/news/ newsLetter/2006/advocate1206.html#1

6. Valeant Pharmaceuticals. "Valeant Pharmaceuticals presents final analyses of Viramidine Phase 2 clinical trial at EASL; Viramidine Phase 2 SVR data presented in detail; Four Valeant abstracts accepted for presentation at EASL." *Business Wire*. April, 2005. www.findarticles.com/p/articles/mi_m0EIN/is _2005_April_18/ai_n13628092

    Watson, J. "Prospects for hepatitis C virus therapeutics: levovirin and viramidine as improved derivatives of ribavirin." *PubMed*. May 2003. www.ncbi.nlm.nih.gov/entrez/query.fcgi?cmd=Retrieve&db=PubMed&list_uids= 12090539&dopt=Abstract

    Baker, Ronald Ph.D. "Hepatitis C drug Viramidine fails pivotal Phase III trial, again." HIVandHepatitis.com, 2006. www.hivandhepatitis.com/hep_c/news/2006/091506_d.html

    Baker, Ronald Ph.D. "The search for improved treatments for chronic hepatitis C." HIVandHepatitis.com, July 2005. www.hivandhepatitis.com/hep_c/news/2006/091506_d.html

    National Institute of Diabetes and Digestive and Kidney Diseases. "Chronic hepatitis C: current disease management." www.disgestive.niddk.nih.gov/ddiseases/pubs/chronichepc/index.htm

    Amarillo Bioscience. "Low dose oral interferon alpha our lead product." 2006. www.amarbio.com/03productcandidate.html

    Human Genome Sciences. "Albuferon." 2006. www.hgsi.com/products/ albuferon.html

    Intarcia Therapeutics, Inc. "Infectious diseases—omega duros for hepatitis C." 2006. www.intarcia.com/products.html

7. Franciscus, Alan. "Hepatitis C treatments in current clinical development." *HCV Advocate*. Dec. 2006. www.hcvadvocate.org/hepatitis/hepC/HCVDrugs.html

    "New Investigational Vaccine To Prevent Hepatitis C Tested For First Time In Humans." *Science Daily*. Nov. 2003. www.sciencedaily.com/releases/2003/11/031117073403.htm

    Saint Louis University. "The hunt for a hepatitis C vaccine is under way at Saint Louis University School of Medicine." May, 2006. www.slu.edu/readstory/more/6881

    Pevion Biotech. "Hepatitis C vaccine enters clinical phase I." Dec. 2006. www.pevion.com/index.php?section=news&cmd=details&newsid=199& teaserId=20

    Choi, Charles. "The world's first preventative vaccine against Hepatitis C could curb the spread of the disease that killed Allen Ginsberg and thousands of others." *Scientific American*. Dec. 2006. www.sciam.com/article.cfm?articleID=729CC919-E7F2-99DF- 3538AD2FBBA3908C

    Pittman, Asa. "SLU tests vaccine to ward off hepatitis C, liver cancer." *St. Louis Business Journal*. May 2006. stlouis.bizjournals.com/stlouis/stories/2006/ 05/15/focus7.html?from_yf=1

Month 5

1. Steckelberg, James, M.D. "How common is sexual transmission?" Mayo Clinic. www.mayoclinic.com/health/hepatitis-c/AN00701

   Palmer, Melissa, M.D. *Dr. Melissa Palmer's Guide to Hepatitis and Liver Disease: What You Need to Know.* Revised Edition. Avery, 2004, pp. 114–5.

Month 8

1. Alter, M. J. et al. The prevalence of hepatitis C virus infection in the United States, 1988 through 1994. *N Engl J Med.* 1999;341(8):556–62; www.ncbi.nlm.nih.gov/entrez/query.fcgi?db=PubMed&cmd=Retrieve& list_uids=10451460.

2. PKIDs (Parents of Kids With Infectious Diseases). "Hepatitis C in children." *Pediatric Hepatitis Report*, pp. 120. www.pkids.org/pdf/phr/03-01hcv.pdf

   Palmer, p. 113.

3. Bellentani S, Tiribelli C. "The spectrum of liver disease in the general population: lesson from the Dionysos study." *J Hepatol.* 2001;35(4):531–7. gut.bmj.com/cgi/content/full/44/6/874

4. Wiese, M. et al. "Low frequency of cirrhosis in a hepatitis C (genotype 1b) single-source outbreak in germany: a 20-year multicenter study." *Hepatology.* 2000;32(1):91–6. www.ncbi.nlm.nih.gov/entrez/query.fcgi?db=PubMed &cmd=Retrieve&list_uids=10869294.

   Kenny-Walsh E. "Clinical outcomes after hepatitis C infection from contaminated anti-D immune globulin." Irish Hepatology Research Group. *N Engl J Med.* 1999;340(16):1228–33. www.ncbi.nlm.nih.gov/entrez /query.fcgi?db=PubMed&cmd=Retrieve&list_uids=10210705.

5. Howell, C., Jeffers, L., Hoofnagle, J. H. "Hepatitis C in African Americans: summary of a workshop." *Gastroenterology.* 2000;119(5):1385–96. www.ncbi.nlm. nih.gov/entrez/query.fcgi?db=PubMed&cmd=Retrieve&list_uids=11054398.

6. Chen, Stephen L. and Timothy R. Morgan. "The natural history of hepatitis C virus (HCV) infection." *International Journal of Medical Science.* 2006; 3(2): 47–52. www.pubmedcentral.nih.gov/articlerender.fcgi?artid=1415841#top

   Seeff, L. B. et al. "Long-term mortality and morbidity of transfusion-associated non-A, non-B, and type C hepatitis: A National Heart, Lung, and Blood Institute collaborative study." *Hepatology.* 2001;33(2):455–63. www.ncbi.nlm.nih. gov/entrez/query.fcgi?db=PubMed&cmd=Retrieve&list_uids=11172349.

   Villano, S. A. et al. "Persistence of viremia and the importance of long-term follow-up after acute hepatitis C infection." *Hepatology.* 1999;29(3):908–14. www.ncbi.nlm.nih.gov/entrez/query.fcgi?db=PubMed&cmd=Retrieve& list_uids=10051497.

7. Palmer, p. 135.

8. Ibid.

9. Chen, Stephen L. and Timothy R. Morgan. "The natural history of hepatitis C virus (HCV) infection." *International Journal of Medical Science*. 2006; 3(2): 47–52. www.pubmedcentral.nih.gov/articlerender.fcgi?artid=1415841#top

10. Boseley, Sarah. "Scientists on a mission to bring cheap drugs to the world's poorest countries." *The Guardian*, 2007. education.guardian.co.uk/higher/news/story/0,,1981356,00.html

    Tompkins, Charlotte, Nat Wright, and Lesley Jones, Centre for Research in Primary Care. "Impact of a positive hepatitis C diagnosis on homeless injecting drug users: a qualitative study." *British Journal of General Practice*, 2005. www.pubmedcentral.nih.gov/articlerender.fcgi?artid=1463127

    Nyamathi, A., Dixon, E., Robbins, W., Smith, C., Wiley, D., Leake, B., Longshore, D., Gelberg, L. "Risk factors for hepatitis C virus infection among homeless adults." *J Gen Intern Med* 2002; 17(2):134–143. www.pubmedcentral.nih.gov/articlerender.fcgi?artid=1495011

    Alter, M. J. et al. "The prevalence of hepatitis C virus infection in the United States, 1988 through 1994." *N Engl J Med*. 1999;341(8):556–62; www.ncbi.nlm.nih.gov/entrez/query.fcgi?db=PubMed&cmd=Retrieve&list_uids=10451460.

    Gottlieb, Scott. "Hepatitis C infects almost 2% of US population." *BMJ*. 1999 August 28; 319(7209): 535. www.pubmedcentral.nih.gov/articlerender.fcgi?artid=1116430

    Swan, Tracy. "Current challenges in hepatitis C treatment." *Research Initiative/Treatment Action!* Fall 2004. findarticles.com/p/articles/mi_m0EXV/is_2_10/ai_n13650941

11. National HCV Prison Coalition: Hepatitis C Awareness Project. 2006. www.hcvinprison.org/

    "HCV in prisons." *Hepatitis C Awareness News*. Jan/Feb 2006. www.hcvinprison.org/docs/Jan_Feb_06b.pdf

12. Cheung, Ramsey Chi-Man M.D. "Chronic hepatitis C in the Veteran population." *HCV Advocate*. 2003. www.hcvadvocate.org/hcsp/articles/cheung-1.html

    HCVets.com. "The Hepatitis C Epidemic." 2007. www.hcvets.com/

    U.S. Department of Veterans Affairs. "VA hepatitis C prevalence study results and VA hepatitis C program actions: summary." 2006. www.hepatitis.va.gov/vahep?page=prtop01-rs-01

    NATAP. "VA hepatitis C prevalence study results summary and VA hepatitis C program actions." 2004. www.natap.org/2004/HCV/061104_03.htm

    Dominitz, J.,Boyko, E., Koepsell, T., Heagerty, P., Maynard, C., Sporleder, J. VA Cooperative Study Group 488. "Elevated prevalence of hepatitis C infection in users of United States Veterans medical centers." *Hepatology*. January 2005. www.hepatitis.va.gov/pdf/va01-pr/prtop-01/prevalence.pdf

13. CDC. "Prevention of infectious diseases: hepatitis, viral, type C." *Travelers' Health: Yellow Book, Health Information for International Travel 2005-2006*. Chapter 4. www2.ncid.cdc.gov/travel/yb/utils/ybGet.asp?section=dis&obj=hcv.htm&cssNav=browseoyb

CDC. "Recommendations for prevention and control of hepatitis C Virus (HCV) infection and HCV-related chronic disease." *Morbid Mortal Wkly Rep (MMWR)*. 1998; 47(RR-19):1–39.

Immunization Action Coalition. "If you have hepatitis C, which vaccinations do you need?" Item# P4042. www.immunize.org/catg.d/4042hepc.htm.

National Travel Health Network and Centre. Travel health information sheets. www.nathnac.org/travel/factsheets/hep_c.htm#risk

World Health Organization (WHO). "Infectious diseases of potential risk for travelers." Chapter 5 in *International Travel and Health 2005*. whqlibdoc.who.int/publications/2005/9241580364_chap5.pdf

Month 9

1. M. Berenguer, M.D., T.L. Wright, M.D. Department of Veterans Affairs Medical Center, University of California, San Francisco. "Treatment strategies for recurrent hepatitis C after liver transplantation," *Clinical Liver Disease*, 1999 Nov; 3(4): 883–99.

2. Harriet A. Washington. *Living Healthy with Hepatitis C.* (New York: Dell, 2000), p. 234. A.C. Klassen, M.D., D.K. Klassen, M.D., R. Brookmeyer, M.D., R.G. Frank, M.D., K. Marconi, M.D., "Factors influencing waiting time and successful receipt of cadaveric liver transplant in the United States: 1990 to 1992," *Med Care* 1998 Mar; 36(3): 281–94.

Month 10

1'. American Academy of Pediatrics. "Infections Spread by Blood and Body Fluids." In: Pickering LK, Baker CJ, Long SS, McMillan JA, eds. *Red Book: 2006 Report of the Committee on Infectious Diseases.* 27th ed. Elk Grove Village, IL: American Academy of Pediatrics; 2006: 151–3.

PKIDs (Parents of Kids With Infectious Diseases). "Whom to tell and not tell when a child has viral hepatitis." *Pediatric Hepatitis Report,* pp. 357–364. http://www.pkids.org/pdf/phr/10-01whomtotell.pdf

2. American Academy of Pediatrics. "Infections Spread by Blood and Body Fluids," pp. 151–3.

3. PKIDs. "Whom to tell and not tell when a child has viral hepatitis," pp. 357–364.

4. PKIDs. "Standard Precautions," pp. 285.

5. PKIDS. "Disclosing to Our Children: What the HIV Experience Has Taught Us." *Pediatric Hepatitis Report,* pp. 379–384; http://www.pkids.org/pdf/phr/ 10-03disclosingtokids.pdf

6. PKIDS. "Talking to Children." *Pediatric Hepatitis Report,* pp. 365–378. http://www.pkids.org/pdf/phr/10-02talkingabouthep.pdf

PKIDS. "Disclosing to our children," pp. 379–384.

PKIDs. "Standard Precautions," pp. 285–6.

7. Rosenthal, Philip M.D. "Hepatitis C in children: Update 2006," *HCV Advocate Newsletter,* March 2006.
    http://www.hcvadvocate.org/hcsp/articles/hcv_children_2006.html

    Gonzalez-Peralta RP, Kelly DA, Haber B, et al. "Interferon alfa-2b in combination with ribavirin for the treatment of chronic hepatitis C in children: efficacy, safety, and pharmacokinetics." *Hepatology* 2005; 42:1010–8.

    HIVandHepatitis.com. "Interferon with ribavirin is safe and effective for children with chronic hepatitis C."
    http://www.hivandhepatitis.com/hep_c/news/2005/ad/110105_a.html

Month 11

1. Stop AIDS Project, "HIV-AIDS-STD: Defintions,"
    www.stopaids.org/resources/std_info/definitions.html

2. Centers for Disease Control and Prevention. "Coinfection with HIV and Hepatitis C Virus." July 2005.
    www.cdc.gov/hiv/resources/factsheets/coinfection.htm

    "Recommendations for Management of Chronic Hepatitis B and C in HIV Coinfected Patients." HIVandHepatitis.com. April 2006.
    www.hivandhepatitis.com/hiv_hcv_co_inf/2006/041806_a.html

    "Early Antiretroviral Therapy Is the Most Effective Way to Reduce Liver-related Deaths in HIV/HCV Coinfected Patients." HIVandHepatitis.com. January 2007.
    www.hivandhepatitis.com/hiv_hcv_co_inf/2007/012307_a.html

    "Histological Response to Pegylated Interferon plus Ribavirin in HIV-HCV Coinfected Individuals." HIVandHepatitis.com. November 2006.
    www.hivandhepatitis.com/hiv_hcv_co_inf/2006/111006_a.html

    Camino, N., Sheldon, J., Soriano, V. "Update on hepatitis C treatment in HIV-coinfected patients." *Minerva Gastroenterol Dietol.* March 2004; 50(1):67-77.
    www.ncbi.nlm.nih.gov/entrez/query.fcgi?itool=abstractplus&db=pubmed&cmd=Retrieve&dopt=abstractplus&list_uids=15719008

3. J.Reichen, M.D. "Co-infection hepatitis B and C." www.cx.unibe.ch/ikp/lab2.hbhc.html. Reichen, a professor of clinical pharmacology at the University of Berne, briefly summarizes the results of studies on HCV/HBV coinfection. His endnotes provide an exhaustive list of these studies.

For Further Reading

Books on hepatitis C, conventional, complementary and alternative treatments

HERE ARE some books for further reading. Be aware that the most up-to-date information will be available in print and online journals. We discuss some good journals and Web sites in our chapter on "Keeping Up-to-Date and Doing Research" (Month 7), and we list scientific studies and articles in the next section below.

Askari, Fred K. *Hepatitis C, The Silent Epidemic: The Authoritative Guide.* New York: Kluwer Academic/Plenum Publishers, 1999.

Blumenthal, Mark, et al. eds. *The Complete German Commission E Monographs: Therapeutic Guide to Herbal Medicines.* Newton, MA: Integrative Medicine Communications, 1998.

Blumenthal, Mark, Alicia Goldberg, eds. *Herbal Medicine: Expanded Commission E Monographs.* Newton, MA: 2000.

Chevallier, Andrew. *Encyclopedia of Herbal Medicine: The Definitive Reference Guide to 550 Key Herbs and Remedies for Common Ailments.* DK Adult, 2000.

Cohen, Misha Ruth. O.M.D., L.Ac and Robert G. Gish, M.D. with Kalia Doner. *The Hepatitis C Help Book: A Groundbreaking Treatment Program Combining Western and Eastern Medicine for Maximum Wellness and Healing.* New York: St. Martin's Griffin. 2001.

Daniels, Samuel, M.D. and Vernon Williams. *Hepatitis C: The Black Person's Guide.* Hilton Publishing, 2004.

Dolan, Matthew with Iain M. Murray-Lyon, M.D.. *The Hepatitis C Handbook.* Berkeley: North Atlantic Books. 1999.

Everson, Gregory T. and Hedy Weinberg. *Living with Hepatitis C: A Survivor's Guide.* Third Edition. Long Island City, NY: Hatherleigh Press. 2002.

Fugh-Berman, Adriane, M.D. *Alternative Medicine: What Works.* Baltimore: William & Wilkins, 1997.

Gitnick, Gary, ed. *Critical Issues In Gastroenterology.* Baltimore: Williams & Wilkins, 1998.

Gruenwald, Joerg. *The PDR for Natural Medicines.* Third Edition. Thomson Healthcare, 2004.

Hagedorn, C. H. and C. M. Rice, eds. *The Hepatitis C Viruses. Current Topics In Microbiology And Immunology.* 242; Berlin, London: Springer, 2000.

The Hepatitis C Strategic Plan: A Collaborative Approach to the Emerging Epidemic in California. Berkeley: Health & Education Communication Consultants, 2001.

Jeanne, Heather. *The Hepatitis C Cookbook: Easy and Delicious Recipes.* Nashville: Cumberland House, 2004.

Jenkins, Mark. *Hepatitis C: Practical, Medical and Spiritual Guidelines for Living with HCV.* Center City, MN: Hazelden Books, 2000.

Jones, Ramona, C.N.C. and Vonah L. Stanfield. *A Real "Hep" Cookbook.* Shawnee, OK: Nature's Response.

Lau, Johnson Yiu-Nam, ed. Forewords by T. Jake Liang, et al. *Hepatitis C Protocols.* Totowa, NJ: Humana Press, 1998.

Liang , T. Jake and Jay H. Hoofnagle. *Hepatitis C. Biomedical Research Reports.* San Diego: Academic Press, 2000.

Maddrey, Willis C. *Conquering Hepatitis C.* Hamilton, Ontario, Canada: B.C. Decker, 2000.

National Institute of Diabetes and Digestive and Kidney Diseases, National Institutes of Health. *Chronic Hepatitis C: Current Disease Management.* Bethesda, MD: 2000. www.niddk.nih.gov/health/digest/pubs/chrnhepc/chrnhepc.htm

Palmer, Melissa, M.D. *Melissa Palmer's Guide to Hepatitis and Liver Disease: What You Need to Know.* Revised Edition. Avery Putnam Penguin, 2004.

Parents of Kids With Infectious Diseases (PKIDs). *Pediatric Hepatitis Report.* www.pkids.org/dis_hep_phr.php

Parr, Elizabeth. *I'm Glad You're Not Dead: A Liver Transplant Story*. Galveston: Journey Publishing, 2000.

Petro, Beth Ann M. A., Foreword by Emmet Keefe, M.D. *Hepatitis C: A Personal Guide to Good Health*. Berkeley: Ulysses Press, 1997.

Poynard, Thierry. *Hepatitis C Infection: Management and Treatment*. London: Martin Dunitz, 2000.

Reesink, H. W., vol ed. *Hepatitis C Virus*. 2nd, rev. and enl. ed. New York: Karger, 1998.

Turkington, Carol. *Hepatitis C: The Silent Killer*. Lincolnwood, IL: Contemporary Books, 1998.

Washington, Harriet A. *Living Healthy with Hepatitis C: Natural and Conventional Approaches to Recover Your Quality of Life*. New York: Dell, 2000.

Zhang, Qingcai, L.Ac., M.D. *Healing Hepatitis C with Modern Chinese Medicine*. Sino-Med Institute, 2000.

Scientific studies and articles

SCIENTIFIC STUDIES are usually published in periodicals, because research moves at such a fast pace that it is often outdated by the time a book is published. Here is a list of studies, articles, and press releases from pharmaceutical companies that we refer to in the book. We've provided the links for many of them. Most of the studies are on Medline, and you can get free access to the abstracts through medscape.com. If you are interested in reading the full article, you may need to look up the journal in a medical library or ask a doctor to order the article for you.

Alter, M. J. et al. "The prevalence of hepatitis C virus infection in the United States, 1988 through 1994." *N Engl J Med*. 1999;341(8):556–62; www.ncbi.nlm.nih.gov/entrez/query.fcgi?db=PubMed&cmd=Retrieve&-list_uids=10451460.

Anderson, S., Nevins, C. L., Green, L. K., El-Zimaity, H., Anand, B. S. "Assessment of liver histology in chronic alcoholics with and without hepatitis C virus infection." *Digestive Disease Sciences*. 2001 Jul; 46(7):1393–1398.

Amarillo Bioscience. "Low dose oral interferon alpha our lead product." 2006. www.amarbio.com/03productcandidate.html

Association of Healthcare Journalists. "Chronic Illness: Treatment without cure. Can the system cope?" *Covering the Quality of Healthcare: A Resource Guide for Journalists* 2002. www.healthjournalism.org/qualityguide/chapter3.html

Armstrong, L. E. *International Journal of Sport Nutrition and Exercise Metabolism*. 2002.12:189–206.

Baker, Ronald, Ph.D. "Hepatitis C drug Viramidine fails pivotal phase III trial, again." HIVandHepatitis.com. 2006. www.hivandhepatitis.com/hep_c/news/2006/091506_d.html

———. "The search for improved treatments for chronic hepatitis C." HIVandHepatitis.com. July 2005. www.hivandhepatitis.com/ hep_c/news/2006/091506_d.html

Beitia, G., Cobreros, A., Sainz, L., Cenarruzabeitia, E. "MDMA (ecstasy)-induced hepatoxicity; effect on cytosolic calcium signals in isolated hepatocytes," Liver 1999; 19(3):234–41. www.erowid.org/references/refs_view. php?ID=259

Bellentani, S., Tiribelli, C. "The spectrum of liver disease in the general population: lesson from the Dionysos study." *J Hepatol*. 2001;35(4):531–7. gut.bmj.com/cgi/content/full/44/6/874

Berenguer, M., Ferrell, L., Watson, J., Prieto, M., Kim, M., Rayon, M., Cordoba, J., Herola, A., Ascher, N., Mir, J., Berenguer, J., Wright, T. L. "HCV-related fibrosis progression following liver transplantation: increase in recent years." *Hepatology*. 2000 Apr;32(4):673–84.

Berenguer, M., Lopez-Labrador, F. X., Greenberg, H. B., Wright, T. L. "Hepatitis C virus and the host: An imbalance induced by immunosuppression?" *Hepatology*. 2000 Aug;32(2):433–5.

Berenguer, M., Wright, T. L. "Hepatitis C virus in the transplant setting." *Antiviral Therapy*. 1998;3(Suppl 3):125–36.

Berenguer, M., Wright, T.L. "Treatment strategies for recurrent hepatitis C after liver transplantation." *Clinical Liver Disease*. 1999 Nov;3(4):883–99.

Bica, I., McGovern, B., Dhar, R., et al. "Increasing mortality due to end-stage liver disease in patients with human immunodeficiency virus infection." *Clinical Infectious Diseases*. 2001;32:492–7, cited in "Current Review on Hepatitis C Virus in HIV/HCV Coinfection." Written for NATAP by Andrew Talal, M.D., M.P.H., and Ira Jacobson, M.D. www.natap.org/ 2001/jun/current061101.htm

Boseley, Sarah. "Scientists on a mission to bring cheap drugs to the world's poorest countries." *The Guardian*, 2007. education.guardian.co. uk/higher/news/story/0,,1981356,00.html

Brown, P.J., Neuman, M.G. "Digestive Disease Week 2000 conference report: New treatments for chronic hepatitis C." *Canadian Journal of Clinical Pharmacology*. 2001 Summer;8(2):67–71.

Camino, N., Sheldon, J., Soriano, V. "Update on hepatitis C treatment in HIV-coinfected patients." *Minerva Gastroenterol Dietol*. March 2004; 50(1):67–77. www.www.ncbi.nlm.nih.gov/entrez/query.fcgi?itool=abstract plus&db=pubmed&cmd=Retrieve&dopt=abstractplus&list_uids=15719008

Carvalho, M., Carvalho, F., Bastos, M. L. "Is hyperthermia the triggering factor for the hepatoxicity induced by 3,4-methylenedioxymethamphetamine (ecstasy)? An in vitro study using freshly isolated mouse hepatocytes," *Arch Toxicol* 2001; 74:789–93. www.erowid.org/references/refs_view.php?ID=1143

Carvalho, M., Carvalho, F., Remiao, F., de Lourdes Pereira, M., Pires-Das-Neves, R., de Lourdes Bastos, M. "Effect of 3,4-methylenedioxymethamphetamine ('ecstasy') on body temperature and liver antioxidant status in mice: influence of ambient temperature," *Arch Toxicol* 2002; 76(3):166–172. www.erowid.org/references/refs_view.php?ID=1383

Centers for Disease Control and Prevention (CDC). "Coinfection with HIV and Hepatitis C Virus." July 2005. www.cdc.gov/hiv/resources/factsheets/coinfection.htm

———. "Frequently asked questions about hepatitis C." December 2006. 0-www.cdc.gov.mill1.sjlibrary.org/ncidod/diseases/hepatitis/c/faq.htm#1b1

———. "Prevention of infectious diseases: hepatitis, viral, type C." *Travelers' Health: Yellow Book, Health Information for International Travel 2005-2006*. Chapter 4. www2.ncid.cdc.gov/travel/yb/utils/ybGet.asp?section=dis&obj=hcv.htm&cssNav=browseoyb

———. "Recommendations for prevention and control of hepatitis C Virus (HCV) infection and HCV-related chronic disease." Morbid Mortal Wkly Rep (MMWR). 1998; 47(RR–19):1–39. www.cdc.gov/ncidod/diseases/hepatitis/c/plan/index.htm

Chang, M. H. "Mother-to-infant transmission of hepatitis C virus." *Clinical Investigative Medicine* 1996 Oct;19(5):368–72.

Chen, Stephen L. and Timothy R. Morgan. "The natural history of hepatitis C virus (HCV) infection," in *International Journal of Medical Science*. 2006; 3(2): 47–52, www.pubmedcentral.nih.gov/articlerender.fcgi?artid=1415841#top

Cheung, Ramsey Chi-Man, M.D. "Chronic hepatitis C in the Veteran population." *HCV Advocate*. 2003. www.hcvadvocate.org/hcsp/articles/cheung-1.html

Choi, Charles. "The world's first preventative vaccine against Hepatitis C could curb the spread of the disease that killed Allen Ginsberg and thousands of others." *Scientific American*. December, 2006. www.sciam.com/article.cfm?articleID=729CC919-E7F2-99DF-3538AD2FBBA3908C

Collier, J., Chapman, R. "Combination therapy with interferon-alpha and ribavirin for hepatitis C: practical treatment issues." *BioDrugs*. 2001; 15(4): 225–38.

Corrao, G., Arico, S. "Independent and combined action of hepatitis C virus infection and alcohol consumption on the risk of symptomatic liver cirrhosis." *Hepatology*. 1998 Apr;27(4):914–9.

Corrao, G. et al. "The effect of drinking coffee and smoking cigarettes on the risk of cirrhosis associated with alcohol consumption." *European Journal of Epidemiology*. 1994. Dec;10(6): 657–64.

Corrao, G. et al. "Coffee, caffeine, and the risk of liver cirrhosis." *Annals of Epidemiology*, 2001. Oct;11(7): 458–65.

Cox, Audra. "Hepatitis C complicated by morphine withdrawal." *Medical News Today*. 2005. www.medicalnewstoday.com/medicalnews.php? newsid=32798

de Rave, S. "Allocation of donor organs." *Lancet* 1997 Oct 11;350(9084):1107.

Dominitz, J., Boyko, E. , Koepsell, T., Heagerty, P., Maynard, C., Sporleder, J. VA Cooperative Study Group 488. "Elevated prevalence of hepatitis C infection in users of United States Veterans medical centers." *Hepatology*. January 2005. www.hepatitis.va.gov/pdf/va01-pr/prtop-01/prevalence.pdf

Edlin, B. "Prevention and treatment of hepatitis C in injection drug users." *Hepatology*. November 2002. 36(5 Suppl. 1): S210-9. www.pubmedcentral.nih.gov/articlerender.fcgi?artid=1629041

Franciscus, Alan. "Hepatitis C treatments in current clinical development." *HCV Advocate*. December, 2006. www.hcvadvocate.org/hepatitis/ hepC/HCVDrugs.html

Fried, M. W., Shiffman, M., Sterling, R. K., Weinstein, J., Crippin, J., Garcia, G., Wright, T. L., Conjeevaram, H., Reddy, K. R., Peter, J., Cotsonis, G. A., Nolte, F. S. "A multicenter, randomized trial of daily high-dose interferon-alfa 2b for the treatment of chronic hepatitis C: Pretreatment stratification by viral burden and genotype." *American Journal of Gastroenterology*. 2000 Nov;95(11):3225–29.

Gallus, S. et al. "Does coffee protect against liver cirrhosis?" *Annals of Epidemiology*, 2002. Apr;12(3): 202–205.

Ghobrial, R. M., Steadman, R., Gornbein, J., Lassman, C., Holt, C. D., Chen, P., Farmer, D. G., Yersiz, H., Danino, N., Collisson, E., Baquarizo, A., Han, S. S., Saab, S., Goldstein, L. I., Donovan, J. A., Esrason, K., Busuttil, R. W. A 10-year experience of liver transplantation for hepatitis c: analysis of factors determining outcome in over 500 patients [In Process Citation]. Annals of Surgery 2001 Sep;234(3):384–94.

Gish, Robert G. "Future therapies," *HCV Advocate*, Feb. 2006. www.hcvadvocate.org/hcsp/articles/Future_therapies.html

Glue, P., Rouzier-Panis, R., Raffanel, C., Sabo, R., Gupta, S. K., Salfi, M., Jacobs, S., Clement, R. P. "A dose-ranging study of pegylated interferon alfa-2b and ribavirin in chronic hepatitis C." The Hepatitis C Intervention Therapy Group. *Hepatology* 2000 Sep;32(3):647–53.

González-Peralta, R. P., Kelly, D. A., Haber, B., et al. "Interferon alfa-2b in combination with ribavirin for the treatment of chronic hepatitis C in children: efficacy, safety, and pharmacokinetics." *Hepatology* 2005; 42:1010–8.

Gottlieb, Scott. "Hepatitis C infects almost 2% of US population." *BMJ*. 1999 August 28; 319(7209): 535. www.pubmedcentral.nih.gov/ articlerender.fcgi?artid=1116430

Gridelli, B., Perico, N., Remuzzi, G. [Strategies for a greater supply of organs for transplantation] [Strategie per una maggior disponibilita di organi per il trapianto.] *Recenti Prog Med* 2001 Jan;92(1):9–15.

Halasz, R., Sallberg, M., Lundholm, S., Andersson, G., Lager, B., Glaumann, H., Weiland, O. "The GB virus C/hepatitis G virus replicates in hepatocytes without causing liver disease in healthy blood donors." *Journal of Infectious Diseases.* 2000 Dec;182(6):1756–60.

Harris, D. R., Gonin, R., Alter, H. J., Wright, E. C., Buskell, Z. J., Hollinger, F. B., Seeff, L. B. "The relationship of acute transfusion-associated hepatitis to the development of cirrhosis in the presence of alcohol abuse." *Annal of Internal Medicine.* 2001 Jan 16;134(2):120–24.

Hassoba, H. M., Bzowej, N., Berenguer, M., Kim, M., Zhou, S., Phung, Y., Grant, R., Pessoa, M. G., Wright, T. L. "Evolution of viral quasispecies in interferon-treated patients with chronic hepatitis C virus infection." *Journal of Hepatology.* 1999 Oct;31(4):618–27.

HCVets.com. "The hepatitis C epidemic." 2007. www.hcvets.com

Heathcote, E. J., Shiffman, M. L., Cooksley, W. G., Dusheiko, G. M., Lee, S. S., Balart, L., Reindollar, R., Reddy, R. K., Wright, T. L., Lin, A., Hoffman, J., De Pamphilis, J. "Peginterferon alfa-2a in patients with chronic hepatitis C and cirrhosis." *New England Journal of Medicine.* 2000 Dec 7; 343(23): 1673–80.

Heller, T., Auerbach, J., Williams, T., Moreen, T. R., Jazwinski, A; Cruz, B.; Jeurkar, N.; Sapp, R., Guangziang, L., and Liang, T. J. "An in vitro model of hepatitis C virion production." *Proceedings of the National Academy of Sciences,* Vol. 102, No. 7, |pp. 2579–83.

Hepatitis Central. "Novel virus culture system for hepatitis C." Hepatitis C Information Center. February 2007. hepatitis-central.com/mt/archives/2007/02/novel_virus_cul.html

HIVandHepatitis.com. "Early antiretroviral therapy is the most effective way to reduce liver-related deaths in HIV/HCV coinfected patients. January 2007. www.hivandhepatitis.com/hiv_hcv_co_inf/2007/012307_a.html

Herve, S., Riachi, G., Noblet, C., Guillement, N., et al. "Acute hepatitis due to buprenorphine administration." *Eur J Gastroenterol Hepatol.* Oct 2004: 16(10): 1033–7. www.ncbi.nlm.nih.gov/entrez/query.fcgi?cmd=Retrieve&db=PubMed&list_uids=15371928&dopt=Abstract

Highleyman, Liz. "AASLD: Investigational antiviral therapies for hepatitis C." *HCV Advocate Newsletter,* December 2006, www.hcvadvocate.org/news/newsLetter/2006/advocate1206.html#1

Highleyman, Liz. "HCV continues to replicate in the livers of patients with sustained response to therapy." HIVandHepatitis.com. www.hivandhepatitis.com/hep_c/news/2007/121506_b.html

Hirsch, K. R., Wright, T. L. "'Silent killer' or benign disease? The dilemma of hepatitis C virus outcomes." *Hepatology* 2000 Feb;31(2):536–67.

HIVandHepatitis.com. "Histological response to pegylated intefereon plus ribavirin in HIV-HCV coinfected individuals." November 2006. www.hivandhepatitis.com/hiv_hcv_co_inf/2006/111006_a.html

HIVandHepatitis.com. "Inteferon with ribavirin is safe and effective for children with chronic hepatitis C." www.hivandhepatitis.com/hep_c/news/2005/ad/110105_a.html

HIVandHepatitis.com. "Recommendations for management of chronic hepatitis B and C in HIV coinfected patients." April 2006. www.hivandhepatitis.com/hiv_hcv_co_inf/2006/041806_a.html

Ho, Wenzhe, Douglas, Steven D., et al. "Alcohol increases hepatitis C virus in human cells." *Hepatology*, July 2003; 38:1, 57–65; www.niaaa.nih.gov/NewsEvents/NewsReleases/hepatitis.htm

Ho, Wenzhe, Douglas, Steven D. in *Hepatology;* July 2003; 38:1, 57–65; www.niaaa.nih.gov/NewsEvents/NewsReleases/hepatitis.htm

Howell, C., Jeffers, L., Hoofnagle, J. H. "Hepatitis C in African Americans: summary of a workshop." *Gastroenterology*. 2000;119(5):1385–96; www.ncbi.nlm.nih.gov/entrez/query.fcgi?db=PubMed&cmd=Retrieve&list_uids=11054398.

Huang, E. J., Wright, T. L., Lake, J. R., Combs, C., Ferrell, L. D. "Hepatitis B and C coinfections and persistent hepatitis B infections: clinical outcome and liver pathology after transplantation." *Hepatology* 1996 Mar; 23(3): 396–404.

Human Genome Sciences. "Albuferon." 2006. Available at: www.hgsi.com/products/albuferon.html

Immunization Action Coalition. "If you have hepatitis C, which vaccinations do you need?" Item# P4042. www.immunize.org/catg.d/4042hepc.htm.

Intarcia Therapeutics, Inc. "Infectious Diseases—Omega Duros for Hepatitis C." 2006. www.intarcia.com/products.html

Jaeckel, E., Cornberg, M., Wedemeyer, H., Santantonio, T., Mayer, J., Zankel, M., Pastore, G., Dietrich, C., Manfred, Manns, M. P., and the German Acute Hepatitis C Therapy Group. "Treatment of acute hepatitis C with interferon alfa-2b." *New England Journal of Medicine*. November 15, 2001. See www.nejm.org October 1, 2001.

Johnson, C. K. "High Tylenol doses linked to liver woes." Associated Press. July 2006. www.washtimes.com/national/20060704-115220-4848r.htm

Kenny-Walsh, E. "Clinical outcomes after hepatitis C infection from contaminated anti-D immune globulin." Irish Hepatology Research Group. *New England Journal of Medicine*. 1999;340(16):1228–33, www.ncbi.nlm.nih.gov/entrez/query.fcgi?db=PubMed&cmd=Retrieve&list_uids=10210705.

Klassen, A. C., Klassen, D. K., Brookmeyer, R., Frank, R. G., Marconi, K. "Factors influencing waiting time and successful receipt of cadaveric liver transplant in the United States: 1990 to 1992." *Medical Care*, 1998 Mar;36(3):281–94.

Klatsky, A. et al. "Coffee, cirrhosis, and transaminase enzymes." *Archives of Internal Medicine*, June 12, 2006; vol 166: pp. 1190–95.

Lee, Dennis. "Drug induced liver disease." Medicine Net. 2006. www.medicinenet.com/drug_induced_liver_disease/article.htm

Li, Yuan et al. "Morphine enhances hepatitis C (HCV) replicon expression." *American Journal of Pathology*, 2003. 163:1167–75. ajp.amjpathol.org/cgi/content/full/163/3/1167

Lin, O. S., Keeffe, E. B. "Current treatment strategies for chronic hepatitis B and C." *Annual Review of Medicine*. 2001;52:29–49.

Liu, J., Manheimer, E., Tsutani, K., et al. "Medicinal herbs for hepatitis C virus infection: a Cochrane hepatobiliary systematic review of randomized trials." *The American Journal of Gastroenterology*. 2003;98(3):538–44.

Manns, M. P., Cornberg, M., Wedemeyer, H. "Current and future treatment of hepatitis C." *Indian Journal of Gastroenterology*. 2001 Mar;20 Suppl 1:C47–51.

Mauss, S. et al. "A prospective controlled study of interferon-based therapy of chronic hepatitis C in patients on methadone maintenance." *Hepatology*. July 2004. 40 (1): 120–24. www.ncbi.nlm.nih.gov/entrez/query. fcgi?cmd=Retrieve&db=PubMed&list_uids=15239094&dopt=Abstract

Monto, Alexander, et al. "Risks of a range of alcohol intake on hepatitis C-related fibrosis," *Hepatology*, March 2004; 39:3; https://www.aasld.org/eweb/DynamicPage.aspx?webcode=press_release_hep4

Morrill, James A., M.D., Ph.D; Shrestha, M., B.S., CHES, and Grant, Richard W., M.D., MPH. "Barriers to the treatment of hepatitis C: patient, provider, and system factors." *J Gen Intern Med*. 2005 August; 20(8): 754–58. www.pubmedcentral.nih.gov/articlerender.fcgi?artid=1490173

NATAP. "VA hepatitis C prevalence study results summary and VA hepatitis C program actions." 2004. www.natap.org/2004/HCV/061104_03.htm

National Institute of Diabetes and Digestive and Kidney Diseases. "Chronic hepatitis C: current disease management." www.disgestive.niddk.nih.gov/ddiseases/pubs/chronichepc/index.htm

"New in vitro model system will allow study of therapeutics and virus life cycle." Press Release. February 22, 2005. www.niddk.nih.gov/welcome/releases/02-22-05.htm

National Institutes of Health Consensus Development Conference Statement: Management of Hepatitis C 2002 (June 10–12, 2002). *Gastroenterology*. 2002;123(6):2082–99.)

National Travel Health Network and Centre. Travel health information sheets. www.nathnac.org/travel/factsheets/hep_c.htm#risk

Nevins, C.L., Malaty, H., Velez, M.E., Anand, B.S. "Interaction of alcohol and hepatitis C virus infection on severity of liver disease." *Digestive Disease Sciences*.1999 Jun;44(6):1236–42.

Noda K. et al. "Progression of type C chronic hepatitis to liver cirrhosis and hepatocellular carcinoma—its relationship to alcohol drinking and the age of transfusion." *Alcohol Clin Exp Res*. 1996;20(1 Suppl):95A–100A.

Nyamathi, A., Dixon, E., Robbins, W., Smith, C., Wiley, D., Leake, B., Longshore, D., Gelberg, L. "Risk factors for hepatitis C virus infection among homeless adults." *J Gen Intern Med* 2002; 17(2):134–43. www.pubmedcentral.nih.gov/articlerender.fcgi?artid=1495011

Ostapowicz, G., Watson, K.J., Locarnini, S.A., Desmond, P.V. "Role of alcohol in the progression of liver disease caused by hepatitis C virus infection." *Hepatology* 1998 Jun;27(6):1730–35.

Partnership for Solutions. "Better lives for people with chronic conditions." 2001. www.partnershipforsolutions.org

Pessione, F., Degos, F., Marcellin, P., Duchatelle, V., Njapoum, C., Martinot-Peignoux, M., Degott, C., Valla, D., Erlinger, S., Rueff, B. "Effect of alcohol consumption on serum hepatitis C virus RNA and histological lesions in chronic hepatitis C." *Hepatology* 1998 Jun;27(6):1717–22.

Pessoa, M.G., Bzowej, N., Berenguer, M., Phung, Y., Kim, M., Ferrell, L., Hassoba, H., Wright, T. L. "Evolution of hepatitis C virus quasispecies in patients with severe cholestatic hepatitis after liver transplantation." *Hepatology* 1999 Dec;30(6):1513–20.

Pessoa, M. G., Terrault, N. A., Detmer, J., Kolberg, J., Collins, M., Hassoba, H. M., Wright, T. L. "Quantitation of hepatitis G and C viruses in the liver: evidence that hepatitis G virus is not hepatotropic." *Hepatology* 1998 Mar;27(3):877–80.

Peters, M. G, Terrault, N. A. "Alcohol use and hepatitis C." *Hepatology*. 2002;36(5 Suppl 1):S220–25.

Pevion Biotech. "Hepatitis C vaccine enters clinical phase I." Dec. 2006. www.pevion.com/index.php?section=news&cmd=details& newsid=199&teaserId=20

Pittman, Asa. "SLU tests vaccine to ward off hepatitis C, liver cancer." *St. Louis Business Journal*. May 2006. stlouis.bizjournals.com/ stlouis/stories/2006/05/15/focus7.html?from_yf=1

Poynard, T., Bedossa, P., Opolon, P. "Natural history of liver fibrosis progression in patients with chronic hepatitis C." The OBSVIRC, METAVIR, CLINIVIR, and DOSVIRC groups. *Lancet*. 1997;349(9055):825–32.

Reddy, K. R., Wright, T. L., Pockros, P. J., Shiffman, M., Everson, G., Reindollar, R., Fried, M. W., Purdum, P. P., Jensen, D., Smith, C., Lee, W. M., Boyer, T. D., Lin, A., Pedder, S., De Pamphilis, J. "Efficacy and safety of pegylated (40-kd) interferon alpha-2a compared with interferon alpha-2a in noncirrhotic patients with chronic hepatitis C." *Hepatology* 2001 Feb;33(2):433–38.

Rosenthal, Philip, M.D. "Hepatitis C in children: update 2006." *HCV Advocate Newsletter*. March 2006. www.hcvadvocate.org/hcsp/ articles/hcv_children_2006.html

Saint Louis University. "The hunt for a hepatitis C vaccine is under way at Saint Louis University School of Medicine." May 2006. www.slu.edu/ readstory/more/6881

Seeff L. B. et al. "Long-term mortality and morbidity of transfusion-associated non-A, non-B, and type C hepatitis: A National Heart, Lung, and Blood Institute collaborative study." *Hepatology.* 2001;33(2):455–63; www.ncbi.nlm.nih.gov/entrez/query.fcgi?db=PubMed&cmd=Retrieve&list_uids=11172349

Shiffman, M. L. "Pegylated interferons: what role will they play in the treatment of chronic hepatitis C?" *Current Gastroenterology Reports.* 2001 Feb;3(1):30–37.

Simmonds, P. "Viral heterogeneity of the hepatitis C virus." *Journal of Hepatology.* 1999;31 Suppl 1:54–60.

Smith, V. J. R.N., B.S.N., M.A. "How durable is the HCV sustained viral response?" National AIDS Treatment Advocacy Project (NATAP). August 2004. www.natap.org/2004/HCV/083004_06.htm

Steckelberg, James, M.D., "How common is sexual transmission?" Mayo Clinic, www.mayoclinic.com/health/hepatitis-c/AN00701

Sylvestre, D.L. "Treating hepatitis C in methadone maintenance patients: an interim analysis." *Drug Alcohol Depend.* July 2002. 67(2): 117–23. www.ncbi.nlm.nih.gov/entrez/query.fcgi?cmd=Retrieve&db=PubMed&list_uids=12095661&dopt=Abstract

Tompkins, Charlotte, Wright, Nat, and Jones, Lesley. Centre for Research in Primary Care. "Impact of a positive hepatitis C diagnosis on homeless injecting drug users: a qualitative study." *British Journal of General Practice,* 2005. www.pubmedcentral.nih.gov/articlerender.fcgi?artid=1463127

Trocho, C. "The Barcelona Report." www.presidiotex.com/barcelona/

UIC College of Pharmacy. "Use of pain medications in hepatic insufficiency." www.uic.edu/pharmacy/services/di/liver.htm

U.S. Census Bureau. "Income, Poverty and Health Insurance Coverage in the United States: 2004." August 2005. www.census.gov/prod/2005pubs/p60-229.pdf

U.S. Department of Labor. "Health Plans and Benefits." January 2007. www.dol.gov/dol/topic/health-plans/index.htm

U.S. Department of Veterans Affairs. "VA hepatitis C prevalence study results and VA hepatitis C program actions: summary." 2006. www.hepatitis.va.gov/vahep?page=prtop01-rs-01

Valeant Pharmaceuticals. "Valeant Pharmaceuticals Presents Final Analyses of Viramidine Phase 2 Clinical Trial at EASL; Viramidine Phase 2 SVR Data Presented in Detail; Four Valeant Abstracts Accepted for Presentation at EASL." *Business Wire.* April, 2005. www.findarticles.com/p/articles/mi_m0EIN/is_2005_April_18/ai_n13628092

Verrando, R., Robaeys G., Mathei C., Buntinx F.. "Methadone and buprenorphine maintenance therapies for patients with hepatitis C virus infected after intravenous drug use." *Acta Gastroenterol Belg.* Jan–Mar, 2005:

68(1):81–85. www.ncbi.nlm.nih.gov/entrez/query.fcgi?cmd= Retrieve&db=PubMed&list_uids=15832591&dopt=Abstract

Villano, S. A. et al. "Persistence of viremia and the importance of long-term follow-up after acute hepatitis C infection." *Hepatology.* 1999;29(3):908–14; www.ncbi.nlm.nih.gov/entrez/query.fcgi?db=PubMed&cmd= Retrieve&list_uids=10051497.

Waldrep, T. W., Summers, K.K., Chiliade, P.A. "Coinfection with HIV and HCV: more questions than answers?" *Pharmacotherapy* 2000 Dec;20(12):1499–507.

Watson, J. "Prospects for hepatitis C virus therapeutics: levovirin and virami-dine as improved derivatives of ribavirin." May 2003. www.ncbi.nlm.nih.gov/entrez/query.fcgi?cmd=Retrieve&db=PubMed&list _uids=12090539&dopt=Abstract

Wiese, M. et al. "Low frequency of cirrhosis in a hepatitis C (genotype 1b) single-source outbreak in germany: a 20-year multicenter study." *Hepatology.* 2000;32(1):91–96; www.ncbi.nlm.nih.gov/entrez/query. fcgi?db=PubMed&cmd=Retrieve&list_uids=10869294.

Wiley T. E. et al. "Impact of alcohol on the histological and clinical progres-sion of hepatitis C infection." *Hepatology.* 1998;28(3):805–809.

World Health Organization (WHO). "Infectious diseases of potential risk for travelers," Chapter 5 in *International Travel and Health 2005.* whqlibdoc.who.int/publications/2005/9241580364_chap5.pdf

Zhou, S., Terrault, N. A., Ferrell, L., Hahn, J. A., Lau, J. Y., Simmonds, P., Roberts, J. P., Lake, J. R., Ascher, N.L., Wright, T. L. "Severity of liver dis-ease in liver transplantation recipients with hepatitis C virus infection: rela-tionship to genotype and level of viremia." *Hepatology* 1996 Nov;24(5):1041–46.

Zignego, A. L., Fontana, R., Puliti, S., Barbagli, S., Monti, M., Careccia, G., Giannelli, F., Giannini, C., Buzzelli, G., Brunetto, M. R., Bonino, F., Gentilini, P. "Relevance of inapparent coinfection by hepatitis B virus in alpha interferon-treated patients with hepatitis C virus chronic hepatitis." *Journal of Medical Virology.* 1997 Apr;51(4):313–318.

Zylberberg, H., Pol, S. "Characteristics and treatment of hepatitis C virus infection in HIV-coinfected subjects." *AIDS Patient Care STDS* 1998 Jan;12(1):11–19.

Conference papers

Afdhal, Nezam H. "Therapy for Hepatitis C." American Association for the Study of Liver Diseases. 51st Annual Meeting and Postgraduate Course. Day 1— October 27, 2000.

Boyle, Brian. "Pegasys plus ribavirin appears superior to rebetron combination ther-apy for chronic HCV." Selected highlights from *Digestive Disease Week 2001*

(DDW 2001). May 20–23, 2001, Atlanta, Georgia. www.hivandhepatitis. com/2001conf/ddw2001/main.html

Fried Michael W., et al. "Pegylated (40 kDa) interferon alfa-2a (PEGASYS) in combination with ribavirin: Efficacy and safety results from a Phase III, randomized, actively-controlled, multicenter study." Abstract 289. AASLD Presidential Plenary session. May 22, 2001.

National Institutes of Health Consensus Development Conference Statement: Management of hepatitis C 2002 (June 10–12, 2002). *Gastroenterology.* 2002;123(6):2082–99.

Reddy, K. Rajender. "Symposium on treatment of chronic hepatitis C: Optimizing patient management with new approaches." Selected highlights from *Digestive Disease Week 2001* (DDW 2001). May 20–23, 2001, Atlanta, Georgia. www.hivandhepatitis.com/2001conf/ddw2001/main.html

Siddiqui, F. et al. "Biochemical, histological and clinical comparisons between African-American and Caucasian patients with chronic hepatitis C in an urban clinic population." Abstract 1877. Selected highlights from *Digestive Disease Week 2001* (DDW 2001). May 20–23, 2001, Atlanta, Georgia. www.hivandhepatitis.com/2001conf/ddw2001/main.html

Resources

Nonprofit/support organizations

American Liver Foundation (ALF)
1425 Pompton Avenue
Cedar Grove, NJ 07009-1000
800-GO-LIVER (465-4837)
800-4-HEP-ABC (443-7222)
www.liverfoundaton.org

Children's Liver Alliance, Australia
23 Dirkala Street
Mansfield Qld 4122, Australia
011-61 7 3219 2864
cla@liverkids.org.au
www.liverkids.org.au/

Children's Liver Disease Foundation
www.childliverdisease.org

HCV Advocate
Hepatitis C Support Project
alanfranciscus@hcvadvocate.org
www.hcvadvocate.org

Hep C Advocate Network
contactus@hepcan.org
www.hepcan.org

Hep-C Alert
660 NE 125th Street
N. Miami, FL 22161
877-HELP4HEP
866-4HEPHIV
www.hep-c-alert.org

Hep C Connection
190 E. 9th Ave, Suite 320
Denver, CO 80203
800-390-1202
www.hepc-connection.org

HepatitisActivist.org
Advocacy@hepatitisactivist.org
www.hepatitisactivist.org

Hepatitis B Foundation
3805 Old Easton Rd
Doylestown, PA 18902
215-489-4900
Fax: 215-489-4313
info@hepb.org
www.hepb.org

Hepatitis C Action & Advocacy Coalition
530 Divisadero St. #162
San Francisco, CA 94117
HAAC_SF@hotmail.com

Hepatitis C Caring Ambassadors
P.O. Box 1748
Oregon City, OR 97045
503-632-9032
Fax: 503-632-9031
lorren@hepcchallenge.org
www.hepcchallenge.org

Hepatitis C Outreach Project
info@hcop.org
www.hcop.org

Hepatitis C Society of Canada
P.O. Box 33544
50 Dundurn Street South
Hamilton, ON, Canada L8P 4X4
800-652-HepC
www.hepatitiscsociety.com

Hepatitis Education Project
4603 Aurora Ave. North
Seattle, WA 98103-6513
206-732-3011
hep@scn.org
www.scn.org/hepatitis

Hepatitis Foundation International (HFI)
504 Blick Drive
Silver Spring, MD 20904-2901
800-891-0707, or
301-622 4200
www.hepfi.org

Hepatitis C Latino Organization
Spanish-language info on Hep C
www.chasque.apc.org/freno/hepcespa.html

Hepatitis Research Foundation
553 Salt Point Turnpike
Poughkeepsie, NY 12601
845-485-7899
845-471-2253
www.heprf.org

HIVandHepatitis.com
www.HIVandHepatitis.com

Latino Organization for Liver Awareness (LOLA)
Debbie Delgado-Vega
P.O. Box 842
Throgs Neck Station
Bronx, NY 10465
888-367-LOLA
Fax: 718-918-0527
www.lola-national.org

Liver Hope
Pat Buchanan
16807 Canterbury Dr
Minnetonka, MN 55345
www.liverhope.com

Parents of Kids with Infectious Diseases (PKIDS)
360-695-0293
Toll-Free: 877-557-5437
www.pkids.org

United Network for Organ Sharing (UNOS)
888-894-6361
www.unos.org

United Liver Association
11646 West Pico Blvd
Los Angeles, CA 90064
310-445-4204

Government agencies

Centers for Disease Control and Prevention
1600 Clifton Road
Atlanta, GA 30333
CDC Hepatitis Hotline
888-443-7232
CDC Public Inquiries: 800-311-3435
www.cdc.gov/ncidod/diseases/hepatitis/

Department of Public Health
For information about hep C in your state, call your State Department of Public Health, Epidemiology Division.

Department of Justice
Disability Rights Section
950 Pennsylvania Ave, NW
Washington, DC 20530
202-514-2000
www.usdoj.gov
Equal Opportunity Employment
Commission (EEOC) and the American
Disabilities Act (ADA)
www.eeoc.gov

NCCAM, National Institutes of Health
9000 Rockville Pike
Bethesda, Maryland 20892 USA
888-644-6226
Fax: 866-464-3616
www.nccam.nih.gov
nccam.nih.gov/health/hepatitisc

**National Digestive Diseases
Information Clearinghouse**
2 Information Way
Bethesda, MD 20892-3570
800-891-5389
Fax: 703-738-4929
digestive.niddk.nih.gov/

National Institutes of Health (NIH)
The largest biomedical research center in
the world. The research arm of the Public
Health Service, U.S. Department of
Health and Human Services. Below are
the institutes that conduct and support
research on hepatitis viruses.

National Institutes of Health
9000 Rockville Pike, Bethesda, MD
20892
301-496-4000
www.nih.gov

**National Institute of Allergy and
Infectious Diseases (NIAID)**
NIAID Office of Communications and
Public Liaison
6610 Rockledge Drive, MSC 6612
Bethesda, MD 20892-6612
301-496-5717
www.niaid.nih.gov

**National Institute of Diabetes &
Digestive & Kidney Diseases (NIDDK)**
National Digestive Diseases Information
Clearinghouse (NDDIC)
2 Information Way
Bethesda, MD 20892-3570
www.niddk.nih.gov

Transplant organizations and agencies

**TransWeb Organ Transplantation
Information Site**
Eleanor Jones
The Northern Brewery, Suite 201
1327 Jones Drive
Ann Arbor, MI 48105
734-998-7314
www.transweb.org

**Transplant Recipients International
Organization, Inc. (TRIO)**
2100 M Street, NW, #170-353
Washington, DC 20037-1233
800-TRIO-386
202-293-0980
www.trioweb.org

**United Network for Organ Sharing
(UNOS)**
804-330-8500
888-894-6361
www.unos.org

**U.S. Department of Health and
Human Services**
Division of Transplantation
888-ASK-HRSA
www.organdonor.gov

Family issues

Children's Liver Alliance, Australia
23 Dirkala Street
Mansfield Qld 4122, Australia
011-61 7 3219 2864
cla@liverkids.org.au
www.liverkids.org.au/

Children's Liver Disease Foundation
www.childliverdisease.org

Parents of Kids with Infectious Diseases (PKIDS)
360-695-0293
Toll-Free: 877-557-5437
www.pkids.org

The Well Spouse Foundation
www.wellspouse.org

Support groups

Hepatitis Newsgroup
USENET sci.med.diseases.hepatitis

HEPV-L
To subscribe, send an email to list-serv@sjuvm.stjohns.edu and type SUBSCRIBE HEPV-L<YOUR FULL NAME> in the body of the email message.

Hepatitis-central.com
(Lists worldwide support groups as well.)
http://hepatitis-central.com/hcv/support/main.html

Hep C Palace
www.heppalace.net/

HepCPrimer.com
www.hepcprimer.com/patient/support.html

Janis & Friends Hepatitis C Support Site
http://janis7hepc.com/our_chat_room_and_message_boards.htm

Objective Medicine
www.objectivemedicine.com (See section on support groups.)

Priority Healthcare Corporation
www.hepatitisneighborhood.com

Information & internet resources

Academic search engines
www.academicinfo.net

Agency for Healthcare Research & Quality
www.ahrq.gov/consumer/diaginfo.htm

Allied Vaccine Group
www.vaccine.org

Alternative Hope for Hep C
877-367-9875
alternativehopeforhepc.com

American Association for the Study of Liver Diseases
hepar-sfgh.ucsf.edu
www.aasld.org

Americans with Disabilities Act
Information Line
800-514-0301 (voice)
800-514-0383 (TDD)

AmericasDoctor.com
www.americasdoctor.com

Ask Doc Misha
(Chinese medicine)
www.docmisha.com

Andrew Weil, M.D.
www.drweil.com

Ask Jeeves
www.askjeeves.com

The Canadian Liver Foundation
www.liver.ca

CDC Emerging Diseases Page
www.cdc.gov/ncidod/eid/index.htm

CenterWatch Clinical Trials Listing Service
www.centerwatch.com

Information on clinical trials
www.clinicaltrials.com

Columbia University Diseases of the Liver
www.cumc.columbia.edu/dept/medicine/divisions/gi/disliv.html

Consumer Labs
1 North Broadway, 4th Floor
White Plains, NY 10601
914-289-1670
www.consumerlab.com

Dr. Melissa Palmer's Home Page
www.liverdisease.com

Dr. C. Everett Koop: the Web site of the former Surgeon General
www.Epidemic.org

Online Encyclopedias
Search Columbia Encyclopedia or Gray's Anatomy: www.bartleby.com
Encyclopedia Britannica:
www.britannica.com

FDA: up-to-date information on which drugs have been approved by the FDA
www.fda.gov/cder/da/da.htm

HCVadvocate.org

Health Concerns
www.HealthConcerns.com/pro

HealthGrades.com
www.healthgrades.com

Hepatitis B Information and Support List
www.geocities.com/Heartland/Estates/9350/hblist.html

HepatitisActivist.org: provides prewritten letters for your Representatives

Hep-C ALERT!: a nonprofit hepatitis advocacy organization
www.hep-c-alert.org

Hepatitis C Society
www.hepatitiscsociety.com

Hepatitis Central
www.hepatitis-central.com

Hep C Primer
www.HepCPrimer.com

Hep C Vets
hepcvets.com
www.hcvets.com

Hepatitis Directory of On-line Resources:
www.objectivemedicine.com/dbsearch.htm

HepNet—The Hepatitis Information Network
A source for both doctors and patients about viral hepatitis
www.hepnet.com

Hepatitis Neighborhood
250 Technology Park, #124
Lake Mary, FL 32746
800-892-9622
www.hepatitisneighborhood.com

Hepatology Watch
Emmet B. Keefe
Chair of the Editorial Board
www.hepwatch.com

HIV and Hepatitis.com
www.hivandhepatitis.com

Merck Manual of Medical Information-Home Edition
www.merckhomeedition.com

MEDLINE, US National Library of Medicine (NLM)
World's largest database of medical literature
You can get free access to MEDLINE through the following sites:
www.medscape.com
www.ncbi.nlm.nih.gov/pubmed
www.pubmedcentral.nih.gov

Medscape
www.medscape.com

Natap.org: latest information on coinfection
www.natap.org

National Digestive Diseases Information Clearinghouse
2 Information Way
Bethesda, MD 20892-3570
301-654-3810
Fax: 301-907-8906
digestive.niddk.nih.gov/

National HCV in Prison
PO Box 41803
Eugene, OR 97404
541-607-5725
Fax: 541-607-5684
www.hcvinprison.org

National Hepatitis-c.org
www.nationalhepatitis-c.org

Veterans Helping Veterans
www.geocities.com/Pentagon/Bunker/2704

WebMD
www.webmd.com

Whole HealthMD
632 Broadway, 5th Floor
New York, NY 10012
www.wholehealthmd.com

Complementary and alternative treatments/ medical associations

American Art Therapy Association
www.arttherapy.org/

American Association of Oriental Medicine
PO Box 162340
Sacramento, CA 95816
866-455-7999
Fax: 916-443-4766
www.aaom.org

American Association of Naturopathic Physicians
4435 Wisconsin Ave NW Suite 403
Washington, DC 20016
Toll free: 866-538-2267
Local: 202-237-8150
Fax: 202-237-8152
www.naturopathic.org

American Association for the Study of Liver Diseases
www.aasld.org

American Botanical Council
www.herbalgram.org

American Gastroenterological Association
4930 Del Ray Avenue
Bethesda, MD 20814
301-654-2055
Fax: 301-654-5920
www.gastro.org

American Herbalists Guild
141 Nob Hill Road
Cheshire, CT 06410
203-272-6731
www.americanherbalistsguild.com

American Holistic Medical Association
PO Box 2016
Edmonds, WA 98020
425-967-0737
Fax: 425-771-9588
www.holisticmedicine.org

American Medical Association
515 North Street 515 N. State Street
Chicago, IL 60610
800-621-8335
www.ama-assn.org/aps/amahg.htm

HealingPeople.com
Lists acupuncturists and healers across the country
www.healingpeople.com

Health Concerns
510-639-0280
Fax: 510-639-9140
www.HealthConcern.com/pro

Herb Research Foundation
303-449-2265
www.herbs.org

**International Academy of
Compounding Pharmacists**
800-927-IACP (4227)
www.iacprx.org

Marijuana Policy Project
P.O. Box 77492
Capitol Hill
Washington, D.C. 20013
202-462-5747
www.mpp.org

**National Association of Boards of
Pharmacy (NABP)**
1600 Feehanville Drive
Mount Prospect, IL 60056
847-391-4406
www.nabp.net

**National Center for Complementary
and Alternative Medicine (NCCAM)**
National Institutes of Health
9000 Rockville Pike
Bethesda, Maryland 20892 USA
888-644-6226
Fax: 866-464-3616
www.nccam.nih.gov
nccam.nih.gov/health/hepatitisc

**National Certification Commission of
Acupuncture**
703-548-9004
www.nccaom.org

Paths to Wholeness
Misha R. Cohen, OMD, L.A.c
415-864-7234
www.docmisha.com

Quan Yin Healing Arts Center
455 Valencia St
San Francisco, CA 94103-3416
415-861-4964
www.quanyinhealingarts.org

Wei de Ren, M.D.
Traditional Chinese Herbal Treatment for
Hepatitis & HIV Infection
www.dr-ren.com

Vitamin Research Products Inc.
4610 Arrowhead Drive
Carson City, NV 89706
800-877-2447
www.vrp.com

WebMD
www.webmd.com

Andrew Weil, M.D.
www.drweil.com

Whole HealthMD
46040 Center Oak Plaza, Suite 130
Sterling, VA 20166
www.wholehealthmd.com

Zhang's Clinic
420 Lexington Ave, #631
New York, NY 10170-0632
212-573-9584
www.dr-zhang.com/

Conventional treatment/ financial help for drug therapy

Valeant Pharmaceuticals
www.infergen.com
877-361-2719
Infergen Aspire
24/7 Nursing Support and
Reimbursement Program
888-MOVE-FWD

"Be in Charge" Program
Schering Oncology Biotech
888-437-2608
www.beincharge.com

**CenterWatch Clinical Trials Listing
Service**
www.centerwatch.com

Information on clinical trials
www.clinicaltrials.com

FDA: up-to-date information on which
drugs have been approved by the FDA
www.fda.gov/cdeer/da/da.htm

Federal Hill-Burton Free Care Program
5600 Parklawn Bldg., Room 10C-16
Rockville, MD 20857
800-638-0742
Bureau of Primary Health Care
301-594-4100

Finance, Disability and Insurance
National Committee for Quality
Assurance 800-839-6487
Job Accommodation Network
800-232-9675
Social Security
800-772-1213

Glaxo Wellcome Inc
919-248-2100
www.gsk.com/

Hepatitis C Check
Home Access Health (home Hep C test)
800-448-8378
www.homeaccess.com

HepCare
Call Caremark Connect(tm)
800-237-2767
www.hepcare.com

The Medicine Program
www.themedicineprogram.com/

Paths to Wholeness
Misha R. Cohen, OMD, L.A.c
415-864-7234
www.docmisha.com

PegIntron (Schering Plough's pegylated interferon)
www.PegIntron.com
888-437-2608

Ribavirin
www.nlm.nih.gov/medlineplus/druginfo/u
spdi/202509.html
www.hepatitis-central.com/hcv/
ribavirin/toc.html

Hoffman-LaRoche
www.roche.com/home/diseases/dis_
hep.htm
www.pegasys.com
PegAssist is the Pegasys information
program
877-PEG-ASYS (734-2797)

Schering-Plough's Commitment to Care Program
Sliding Scale Program
800-521-7157

WebMD
www.webmd.com

Whole HealthMD
46040 Center Oak Plaza, Suite 130
Sterling, VA 20166
www.wholehealthmd.com

Information for travelers/ healthcare abroad

Healthcare Abroad
243 Church Street West
Vienna, VA 22180
800-237-6615

The International Association for Medical Assistance to Travelers
1623 Military Rd. #279
Niagara Falls, NY 14304-1745
716-754-4883
www.iamat.org/

International SOS Assistance
P.O. Box 11568
Philadelphia, PA 19116
800-523-8930
www.internationalsos.com

Hep C publications

Gastroenterology
The official journal of the American
Gastroenterological Association
subscription fee
www.gastrojournal.org

Hepatitis Magazine (now called *Liver Health Today*)
523 N. Sam Houston Pkwy East
Suite 300
Houston, TX 77060
800-792-6397 ext. 133
Fax: 281-847-5440
www.hepatitismag.com

Hepatitis Weekly
www.holonet./homepage/IH.htm
www.newsrx.com/newsletters/Hepatitis-
Weekly.html
News, research, and articles on hepatitis

Hepatology
Journal of the American Association for
the Study of Liver Diseases
www3.interscience.wiley.com/cgi-bin/
jhome/106570044
www.aasld.org/eweb/DynamicPage.aspx
?Site=AASLD3&-
webcode=HepatologyJournal

Today's Caregiver Magazine
www.caregiver.com

Drug & alcohol resources

Cocaine Anonymous
www.ca.org/

Drug Abuse Information and Treatment Referral Line
National Institute on Drug Abuse
11426 Rockville Pike, Suite 410
Rockville, MD 20852
800-662-4357
800-662-9832 (Spanish)
800-228-0427 (hearing impaired)

Families Anonymous
www.familiesanonymous.org

Lindesmith Center (Harm Reduction)
www.lindesmith.org

Marijuana Policy Project
P.O. Box 77492
Capitol Hill
Washington, D.C. 20013
www.mpp.org

Narcotics Anonymous
World Service Office: 818-773-9999
www.na.org

National Clearinghouse for Alcohol and Drug Information
800-262-2463 800-729-6686
ncadi.samhsa.gov/

Center for Addictive Problems
www.CAPQualitycare.com

Acknowledgments

WE WOULD like to thank our agent, Carol Mann, and our editors, Matthew Lore and Renée Sedliar—we couldn't have done this book without them. We would also like to thank Dave Newman, Debora Munczek, Ph.D., Rachel Resnick, Jim Fitzgerald, Charlotte Abbott, Roz Parr, and Jerry Stahl for their invaluable help and friendship. Thanks to Jess Medina, William Homer, Patricia SanFelipe, Brian Schmeltz, Frank Miles, Eric Clarkson, and the other hep C patients who donated their time and sat through countless interviews and conversations with us. Thanks to Flash Gordon, M.D., Bert Lum, Pharm.D., David Salvage, M.D., Julian Carter, Ph.D., Robert Morgan Lawrence, Ed.D., D.C., Tanuja Goulet, Linden Young, Catherine Poston, Missy Axelrod, Terry Zwigoff, Jennifer Ashby, M.S., L. Ac., Ed.D., Annalee Newitz, Ph.D., Thomas Roche, Anne Marino, Leslie Ellis, and the Aphrodite group, who helped us edit, fact check, or were all-around good friends. A special thank-you to Teresa L. Wright, M.D., for taking the time to write our foreword.

Index